THE
PINK SALT
TRICK RECIPE FOR
WEIGHT LOSS

The Proven 21-Day Morning Reset That Helps You Burn Fat, Flatten Bloat, and Boost Energy—Without Fad Diets or Complicated Plans

EMILY J. HARPER

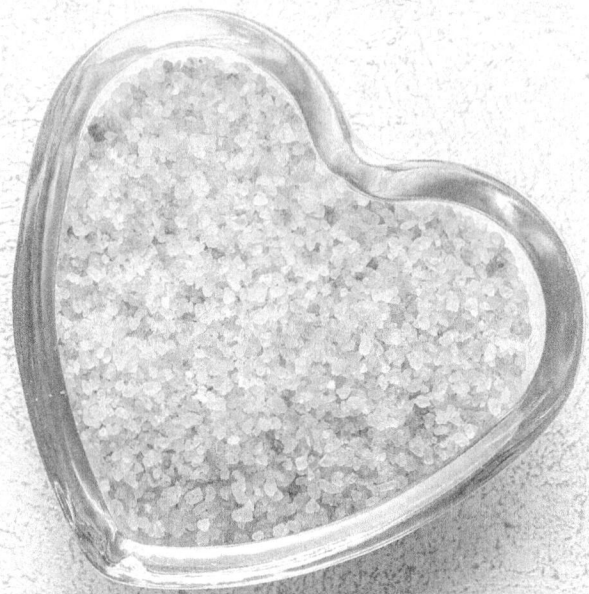

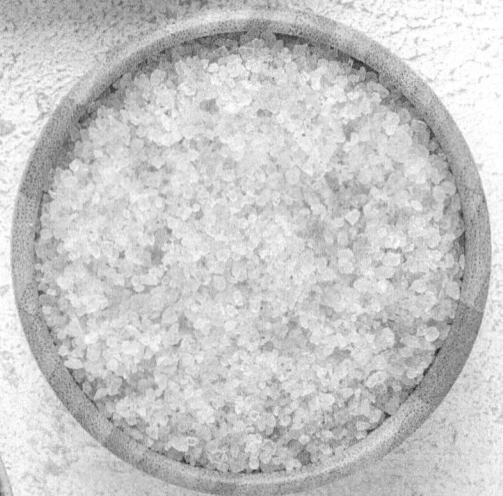

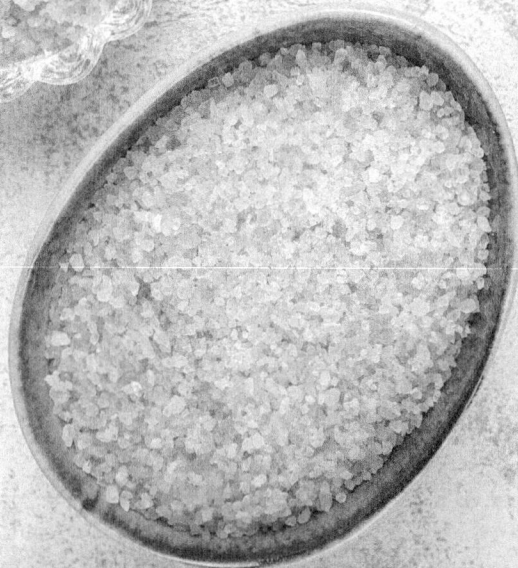

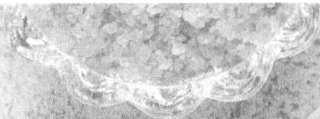

Table of Contents

CHAPTER 5
LUNCH RECIPES

CHAPTER 6
DINNER RECIPES

CHAPTER 7
SNACK RECIPES

CHAPTER 8
TROUBLESHOOTING & FAQS

CHAPTER 9
MAINTENANCE & NEXT STEPS

CONCLUSION

UNLOCK YOUR FREE PINK SALT BONUSES!

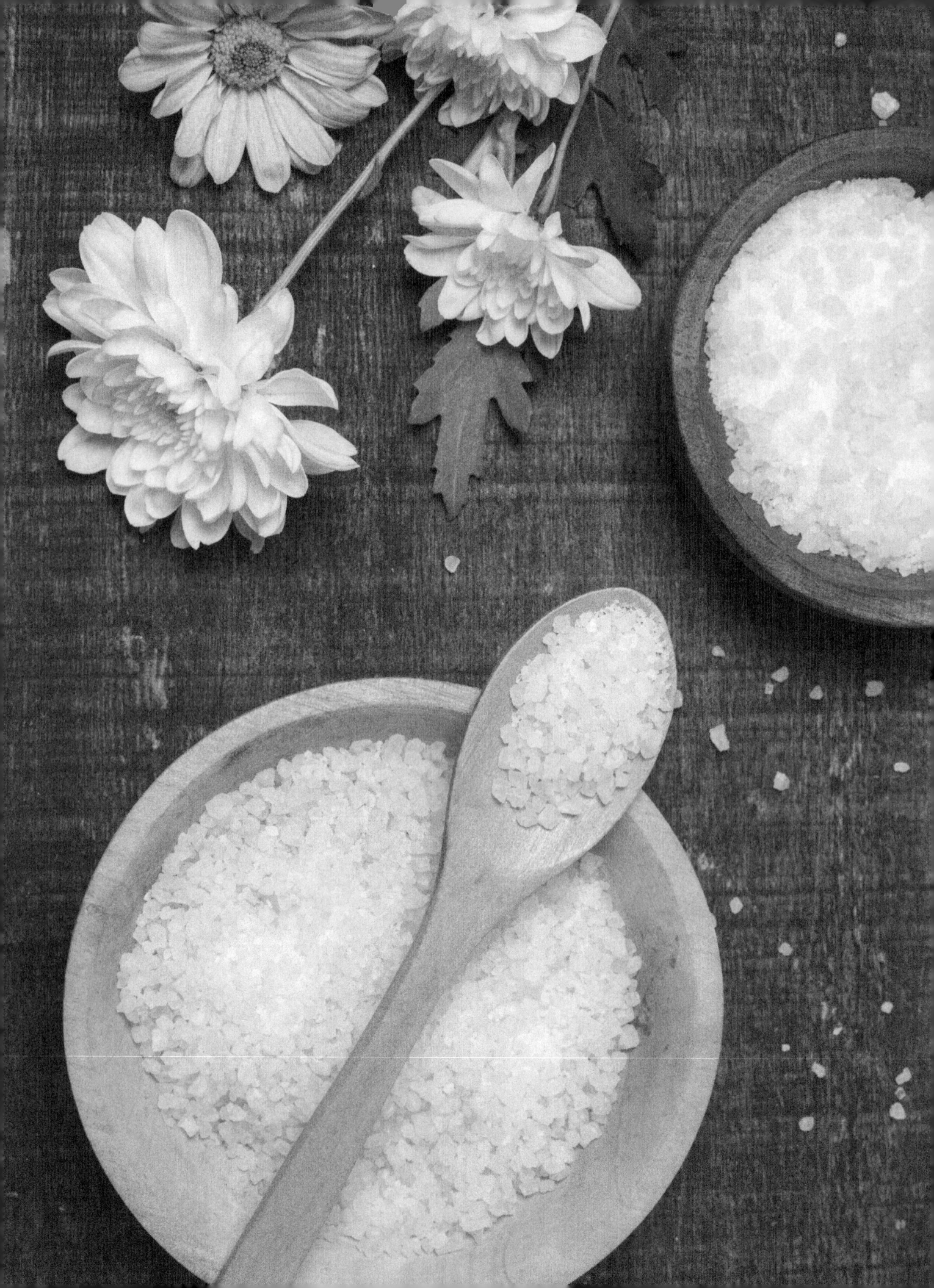

Introduction

UNDERSTANDING THE PINK SALT TRICK

When you first hear about Himalayan pink salt as a tool for weight loss, it might sound too good to be true. After all, salt and diets rarely go hand in hand. Yet this ancient mineral has quietly earned its place in morning routines and wellness circles. Let's unpack what makes pink salt more than just a seasoning—and why adding a simple pinch to your daily ritual can help you feel lighter, more energetic, and ready to tackle the day.

What Sets Himalayan Pink Salt Apart

Not all salts are created equal. Table salt undergoes intense processing: chemicals strip away naturally occurring minerals, leaving nearly pure sodium chloride. In contrast, Himalayan pink salt is harvested from ancient sea beds deep within the mountains of Pakistan. Over millennia, these deposits preserved trace minerals that give the crystals their signature rosy hue and subtle flavor. Among the elements you'll find are calcium, magnesium, potassium, and iron—components that play quiet but important roles in your body's balance.

- Calcium helps muscles contract and relax smoothly.
- Magnesium supports nerve signaling and energy production.
- Potassium regulates fluid balance and blood pressure.
- Iron contributes to healthy red blood cells and stamina.

By choosing pink salt, you're inviting a broader spectrum of minerals into your system—minerals that can influence hydration, digestion, and the tiny electrical currents that keep your cells humming.

How a Pinch of Pink Salt Awakens Your Metabolism

Imagine your body as a finely tuned machine. Every cell depends on electrolytes—minerals that carry an electric charge—to function. When you wake up, you've gone hours without fluid or sustenance. Your cells need a nudge to start their day: signaling muscles, guiding nutrients, and maintaining fluid balance. A morning drink of water with a dash of pink salt delivers that nudge.

- The sodium and potassium in pink salt help your cells draw water back inside after a night of dehydration.
- Better hydration means improved blood flow, which in turn delivers oxygen and nutrients more efficiently.
- With optimum cellular hydration, your digestive system can process food and burn calories more effectively.

You might notice you feel sharper, less sluggish, and more alert soon after adopting this ritual. That's your metabolism responding to better hydration and electrolyte balance—two simple ingredients for a stronger start.

From Tradition to Today's Morning Ritual

People have long turned to mineral-rich springs and salt-infused tonics to support health. In Himalayan villages, salt lamps and salt baths remain common remedies for fatigue and muscle aches. Today, we adapt these traditions for busy lives. Rather than soaking in a tub of pink salt, you stir a quarter teaspoon into eight ounces of warm water first thing each morning. That single act—mixing water, salt, and sometimes a squeeze of lemon—becomes a mindful pause before the day's rush.

Over time, this habit does more than boost hydration. It marks a moment of self-care, a signal to your mind that you're making space for yourself. Many busy parents and professionals report fewer midday crashes, reduced cravings, and a steadier mood when they stick with the ritual.

Backed by Science and Real Experiences

Skepticism is healthy—especially when you've seen one "miracle" drink replace another. While pink salt won't melt fat on its own, researchers have long studied how hydration, electrolytes, and mineral balance affect weight regulation. A 2018 study published in the Journal of Human Nutrition and Dietetics found that properly balanced electrolytes improved participants' exercise performance and recovery, indirectly supporting fat loss over several weeks. During recovery, muscles burn calories more efficiently when not battling mineral imbalances or dehydration.

Meanwhile, real-life case studies bring these findings closer to home. Consider the story of Jessica, a 36-year-old mother of two who struggled with afternoon slump and mindless snacking. She began each day with the pink salt ritual and noticed within a week a sharper appetite control and a natural drop in bloating. By Day 10, she'd lost three pounds and no longer craved sugary treats after lunch.

Customizing Your Pink Salt Drink

There's no one-size-fits-all recipe. Some people find warm water soothing; others prefer it chilled. Here are a few tweaks to help you tailor the drink:

- Warm water with a slice of lemon—gentle on the stomach and adds vitamin C.

- Cool water with a sprig of mint—for a refreshing start on hot mornings.
- A dash of cinnamon or ginger—adds flavor and supports digestion.

Feel free to experiment. The core idea remains the same: you're combining water, a small pinch of mineral-rich salt, and a flavor element that you enjoy. Over days, your body adapts, and you'll come to recognize the subtle lift this ritual provides.

Integrating Pink Salt into Your Day

While the morning drink is the star, pink salt can support other moments too. A pinch on roasted vegetables or in a homemade salad dressing keeps your electrolyte intake steady. For those busy afternoons, a small trail mix with roasted nuts lightly seasoned with pink salt can curb cravings without derailing your progress. Even a brief salt-infused foot soak after a long day can soothe tired muscles and reinforce how this mineral quietly nudges your body toward balance.

Every time you add pink salt to your routine, you remind yourself that healthy habits don't have to be complicated. One simple trick—rooted in tradition, supported by modern insights, and tailored to your life—can become the anchor for better hydration, steadier energy, and a metabolism that works with you rather than against you.

YOUR STARTING POINT: ASSESSING YOUR HEALTH & HABITS

Before you dive into a new ritual or recipe, it helps to know where you stand today. Taking stock of your habits and current health markers gives you a clear checkpoint—and that makes progress feel tangible. You might wonder whether it's worth the time to track these details. Think of it as reading a map before a road trip: you're not lost, but you'll know when you've veered off course.

Charting Your Daily Routine

Your days likely follow a pattern—morning alarms, breakfast routines, work sprints, kid drop-offs, meetings, and evening family time. Each of those moments carries small habits that add up. Notice, for instance, how you hydrate. Do you reach for coffee first thing, only to realize you're already behind on water intake? Or perhaps you rely on sugary snacks to power through the afternoon lull. Jot down your typical day in a simple timeline:

- Wake-up time and first beverage
- Breakfast choices and portion sizes
- Mid-morning snacks or drinks
- Lunch composition, timing, and setting
- Afternoon energy slumps and coping strategies
- Dinner habits, including any treats

- Hydration pattern from morning to bedtime

Seeing this laid out exposes opportunities. Maybe you're dehydrated by mid-morning because coffee outranks water. Or perhaps you skip breakfast on busy days, then over-eat at lunch. These insights guide your tweaks—starting with a morning pink salt drink to reset hydration before caffeine.

Capturing Baseline Metrics

Beyond habits, concrete numbers help you measure change. While the scale tells part of the story, it misses how water, muscle tone, and digestion shift over three weeks. Consider these markers:

- Body weight measured at the same time each morning
- Waist circumference taken at the navel
- Daily energy levels scored on a scale of 1 to 10
- Frequency and quality of your bowel movements
- Sleep duration and restfulness
- Average daily water intake in ounces

You don't need fancy equipment—just a tape measure, a glass, and a journal or app. Track each metric on Day 1, then revisit on Days 7, 14, and 21. Those snapshots reveal trends—perhaps your waist measurement drops even before the scale budges, or you find a more regular digestion pattern by Day 10.

Identifying Habits That Hold You Back

Most of us carry habits that feel harmless but subtly undermine our goals. Maybe you sip soda in the afternoon for a quick pick-me-up, or you mindlessly graze on crackers while checking email. Look for these common slips:

- Relying on caffeinated beverages instead of water between meals
- Eating in front of screens, which can lead to overeating
- Late-night snacking when stress spikes
- Skipping meals and compensating with large portions later
- Ignoring hunger and fullness cues in pursuit of a schedule

Write down when and why these habits occur: is it boredom, stress, or convenience? When you understand the triggers, you can replace them. For example, a pink salt drink may satisfy your mouthfeel craving while delivering electrolytes—no crash later.

Uncovering Hidden Strengths

While you look for stumbling blocks, don't miss the routines that already serve you. Perhaps you take a daily walk after dinner, or you always prepare a balanced lunch on Sundays.

Those actions reflect discipline and foresight—qualities you'll lean on during the 21-day challenge. Note them clearly:

- Existing exercise routines, even short walks
- Meal-prep habits that save time and reduce stress
- Mindful practices like meditation or journaling
- Support systems—friends or family who encourage healthy choices

Emphasizing what you do well builds confidence. When you see that you can plan lunches in advance, you realize creating pink salt recipes won't feel like starting from scratch.

Bringing It All Together

Assessing your health and habits isn't a chore; it's your personalized launchpad. As you fill out your routine, metrics, pitfalls, and strengths, you create a tailored blueprint. Refer back to this data when recipes feel routine or motivation wanes. One evening, you might compare Day 7's hydration tally to Day 1 and realize how much steadier your energy feels. On Day 14, your waist measurement could confirm that this simple morning ritual made a real difference.

Avoid making sweeping changes all at once. Instead, honor small wins. Celebrating your commitment to track water intake or recognizing that you're snacking less sets you up for lasting change. By knowing exactly where you began, you give yourself the gift of clarity—and that makes the path ahead feel far less daunting.

HOW TO USE THIS BOOK FOR MAXIMUM RESULTS

Picking up a new guide can feel like stepping into a vast library—you want to know exactly where to start and how to move through it so you never feel lost. This book is designed to meet you where you are, guiding you through each step of the 21-day pink salt ritual without overwhelming you. To make the most of it, you'll want to set aside a few minutes each morning and evening, gather the simple tools you need, and treat these pages as an interactive manual rather than a one-way lecture.

Finding Your Personal Pace

Everyone's schedule looks different, so before you begin, carve out moments when you can focus. That might be five quiet minutes before the kids wake up or a short break at your desk. Think of these times as your daily appointment with yourself, where you'll stir your pink salt elixir, note how you feel, and review the next steps. If your mornings are tight, consider preparing your salt measure the night before—placing a small container by your bedside or coffee maker so you can grab it without thinking.

At the same time, recognize that life happens. A meeting may run late, or you might have to squeeze in errands. If you miss a morning drink, don't let guilt creep in. Simply pick up again at breakfast or during your mid-morning pause. The key is consistency over perfection. By the end of week one, you'll find it easier to slot this book into your routine.

Making the Chapters Work for You

Rather than reading straight through, treat each chapter like a station on a health track. Here's one way to approach it:

- Scan the chapter summary at the top to see what's ahead.
- Read the core content and highlight tips that speak to your situation.
- Complete any quick exercises—journaling prompts, habit checklists, or hydration logs—before moving on.
- Bookmark or dog-ear pages you want to revisit, such as recipe ideas or troubleshooting tips.

If you find a recipe that matches your taste and schedule, go ahead and try it that day. If a section on habit triggers catches your eye, pause to jot down your own thoughts in the margins or a notebook. This approach turns passive reading into active practice.

Using Recipes as Experiments

The breakfast, lunch, dinner, snack, and drink recipes are not just meal plans; they're experiments you run on yourself. If a lunch bowl feels too heavy on a workday, switch to a lighter recipe and note how your energy shifts. When you try a new shaker blend, record whether it curbs cravings better than your usual snack. Over time, these experiments yield personal data that supplements the baseline metrics you set in the opening chapters.

Tracking Progress and Reflecting

Data doesn't have to be daunting. Think of your notebook or app as a friendly mirror—showing patterns rather than judging them. Setting aside five minutes after dinner to record three things you noticed (level of hunger before dinner, how your morning ritual felt today, any new cravings) helps you tune in to subtle shifts.

- Note how many ounces of water you drank by midday versus your evening glass count.
- Write down your energy scale rating before and after trying a recipe.
- Circle any standout feelings—lighter digestion, steadier focus, or unexpected tiredness.

Every seventh day, flip back to Day 1 entries and compare. You might see that your afternoon slump eased by Day 5 or that you naturally reached for healthier snacks by Day 10. These reflections keep you motivated—showing you real change instead of vague hopes.

Embracing Community and Accountability

Reading a book can feel solitary, but you don't have to go it alone. This guide invites you to connect with others who share the pink salt challenge. You might choose to partner with a friend, swap notes in a private online group, or post daily updates on social media under a tag you create. Hearing about another busy mom who used the recipe to breeze through a long meeting without energy dips can inspire you to stick with the drink—even on days when you'd rather skip it.

If you prefer quiet accountability, consider sharing your Day 1 metrics with someone you trust. Simply telling a spouse or colleague, "I'm starting a three-week ritual and I'll check in on Day 7," adds an external nudge. When you know someone else is aware of your plan, you're more likely to pour that pink salt elixir into your mug before the day takes over.

By treating this book as a living tool—one you use, mark up, revisit, and discuss—you transform it from printed pages into a personalized guide. Each section builds on the last: your baseline informs how you read the recipes; your pace dictates which trouble-shooting tips you consult; your reflections guide the tweaks you make. With this flexible approach, you'll sail through the 21 days with clarity, confidence, and a growing sense that this simple ritual fits neatly into your life.

SETTING SMART GOALS FOR YOUR 21-DAY CHALLENGE

Before you begin stirring your morning pink salt elixir, you need a clear map of what you want to achieve in the next three weeks. SMART goals—Specific, Measurable, Achievable, Relevant, and Time-bound—turn vague wishes into concrete targets. When you set SMART goals for your 21-day ritual, you create checkpoints that guide your actions and help you notice real progress. These aren't lofty declarations; they are down-to-earth objectives you can track each day, keeping you motivated and honest with yourself.

Crafting Specific and Relevant Targets

Specificity transforms "I want to feel better" into "I want to lose 6 pounds and reduce my waist circumference by 2 inches." That level of detail tells you exactly what success looks like. Start by choosing one or two key metrics that matter most to you. As Emily, our busy marketing manager persona, you might focus on energy levels and waist measurements rather than fixating on the scale alone. A goal such as "Increase my average daily energy score from 5 to 7 by Day 14" speaks directly to your desire to keep up with your children and avoid that afternoon crash.

Relevance ensures that your goals align with your lifestyle and values. If you hate the gym but love walking, set a goal tied to steps rather than treadmill miles. By anchoring targets to your personal context—work deadlines, family routines, and preferred activities—you build a plan that feels natural. Ask yourself: what matters most right now? If you struggle with bloating after breakfast, include a goal for digestive comfort, such as "Experience no midday bloating by Day 10."

Ensuring Measurable and Achievable Steps

Measurement turns ambition into data. Without it, you're guessing whether pink salt is helping you or not. Choose metrics that you can record daily with minimal fuss: morning weight, waist circumference, water intake in ounces, and subjective energy ratings on a 1-to-10 scale. These snapshots give you a dimensional view of change. For example, recording eight ounces of pink salt water each morning and noting your energy score before lunch helps you connect cause and effect.

Achievability prevents burnout and disappointment. Losing 6 pounds in three weeks is reasonable for many, but dropping 20 pounds might set you up for frustration. Look at your baseline metrics from earlier chapters and consider small increments. If you currently drink 32 ounces of water daily, aim to reach 64 ounces by Day 7 rather than leaping straight to 100. When in doubt, err on the side of modest targets—you can always raise the bar once you build momentum.

- Specific: "Lose 6 pounds and reduce waist by 2 inches."
- Measurable: "Track weight, waist, water intake, energy levels daily."
- Achievable: "Increase water intake from 32 to 64 ounces by Day 7."
- Relevant: "Boost energy for afternoon school runs without extra caffeine."
- Time-bound: "Reach these targets by the end of Day 21."

Anchoring Goals to Your Timeline

Time-bound goals keep you honest. A 21-day window moves quickly—each day counts. Break your timeline into three seven-day segments, assigning mini-goals for each. In the first week, commit to mastering the pink salt ritual and hydration benchmarks. By Week 2, shift focus to energy scores and morning fullness cues. During the final week, emphasize waist measurements or how many days you avoided sugary snacks after lunch.

Consider crafting a simple chart or using an app that shows Week 1, Week 2, and Week 3 goals side by side. On Day 7, you might aim to have an average energy rating of 6 out of 10 and to have drunk your pink salt water at least five out of seven mornings. On Day 14, you could target a waist measurement reduction of one inch and consistent afternoon hunger control. By Day 21, your SMART goal checklist might read: "Lost 6 pounds, reduced waist by 2 inches, maintained energy rating of 7, and met water intake every morning."

This segmented approach keeps you focused on short-term wins, preventing the overwhelm that comes with aiming only for a three-week outcome. As you mark off each mini-goal, you feel a surge of confidence that propels you into the next phase. And if you miss a checkpoint, the calendar makes it easy to adjust—revisit your targets, identify obstacles, and tweak your plan before moving forward.

By defining precise, measurable targets, ensuring they fit your life, and tying them to a clear timeline, you transform a simple salt ritual into a structured challenge. These SMART goals don't just sit on the page; they become the driving force behind every sip, every recipe you try, and every reflection you record in your journal.

CHAPTER 1

The Science Behind the Pink Salt Trick

HIMALAYAN PINK SALT VS. REGULAR SALT

When you reach for salt at the grocery store, you see white granules in a familiar shaker next to sponges and detergents. That's regular table salt—processed to remove almost everything except sodium chloride. Across the aisle, you might spot a jar of pink crystals that seem to glow with subtle warmth. These are marketed as Himalayan pink salt, an ancient mineral treasure harvested from deep within the Salt Range of Pakistan. The differences between these two salts extend far beyond color and price tag. In this section, you'll learn why choosing pink over white can affect more than taste—impacting hydration, mineral balance, and even the way your body responds to a simple morning ritual.

Origins and Processing Methods

Regular table salt typically begins life as seawater or salt deposits that are pumped from underground wells. The raw crystals undergo heating to evaporate water, followed by bleaching agents to achieve that pristine white appearance. Iodine, introduced in the early 20th century to prevent thyroid problems, is often added back in, as is an anti-caking agent to keep the salt flowing freely.

Himalayan pink salt takes a different path. Formed over 250 million years ago when ancient seas evaporated, the mineral-rich deposits were buried under volcanic lava, protecting them from modern pollution. Miners extract solid rock, then crush and rinse the crystals by hand or machine—no bleaching, no additives. The result is a mosaic of pinks, reds, and grays, reflecting iron oxide and a spectrum of trace minerals. Rather than stripping the salt, this method preserves its natural profile, offering more than just sodium chloride.

Mineral Profiles and Their Effects

At the core, both salts share sodium chloride as their main component—about 97 to 99 percent of each crystal. Yet pink salt carries up to 3 percent of other minerals, depending on the source. That might sound negligible, but those extras influence how your body processes fluids and nutrients throughout the day.

- Calcium—vital for healthy muscle contractions and nerve signals
- Magnesium—supports energy production and muscle relaxation
- Potassium—balances fluids and helps regulate blood pressure
- Iron—contributes to oxygen transport and prevents fatigue
- Zinc—plays a role in immune response and digestion

These minerals work together as electrolytes, carrying electric charges that power cellular functions. When you mix pink salt into water, you're not just adding sodium. You're creating a mild electrolyte solution that can help your cells rehydrate more efficiently after a night without fluids. By contrast, a water-and-table-salt drink delivers primarily sodium, which can cause a temporary fluid shift but lacks complementary minerals to support balanced rehydration.

Taste, Texture, and Culinary Uses

Beyond health, taste and texture come into play. Table salt dissolves instantly, providing a neutral, uniform saltiness. Pink salt's larger crystals take a moment longer to dissolve, delivering gentle bursts of flavor and a subtle crunch if you use it as a finishing salt on salads or roasted vegetables. That tactile difference can turn a simple meal into a sensory experience—encouraging you to slow down, savor each bite, and feel more connected to what you eat.

Chefs and home cooks alike appreciate pink salt for its visual appeal and nuanced flavor. Whereas table salt can taste flat, pink salt carries faint mineral undertones that complement citrus, herbs, and root vegetables without overwhelming delicate dishes. In a morning elixir, you'll notice a softer saltiness that pairs well with a squeeze of lemon or a slice of ginger—making the ritual something you look forward to rather than a chore.

Health Considerations and Myths

Some critics dismiss pink salt as a marketing gimmick—arguing that trace minerals exist only in tiny amounts. They're right that you won't meet your daily magnesium needs by stirring a pinch into water. Yet the role of pink salt is not to replace supplements but to kickstart hydration with a more balanced electrolyte mix. In traditional Himalayan villages, people still believe in salt's healing power—using salt lamps for air quality and salt baths for muscle tension.

Regular table salt, stripped of minerals, can also have drawbacks. Anti-caking agents like sodium aluminosilicate or magnesium carbonate may irritate sensitive digestive tracts in some individuals. Meanwhile, iodized salt can mask other iodine sources in your diet, creating confusion about actual intake levels. If you rely solely on table salt for iodine, you may overlook natural I-rich foods such as seaweed, dairy, and eggs.

Choosing pink salt does come with caution. Because it lacks a universal standard for iodine, relying exclusively on pink salt could risk low iodine intake for those with marginal thyroid function. That's why this book recommends pairing the pink salt ritual with a balanced diet that includes iodine-rich foods or supplements if necessary—especially for anyone who has thyroid concerns or follows a low-sodium medical plan.

Practical Implications for Your Morning Ritual

As Emily, our busy marketing manager persona, you want a simple habit that fits into your morning rush without extra fuss. Swapping table salt for pink salt doesn't add complexity—just open the jar, scoop, and stir. Yet that small change triggers a slightly richer electrolyte mix that can make your first glass of water more satisfying. You're less likely to chase caffeine with more caffeine or crave sugary snacks fifteen minutes later.

Over the first week, pay attention to subtle shifts. You might notice a smoother digestion pattern or a more sustained energy curve between breakfast and lunch. Journal entries that compare how you feel after a plain water start versus a pink salt drink can reveal patterns you never expected. Those observations guide adjustments—for instance, adding a pinch of cinnamon to the mix for a flavor twist that also supports blood sugar balance.

If you ever wonder whether pink salt truly matters, experiment directly. Try a three-day switch: use table salt for one bottle of morning water, then use pink salt for another, while keeping everything else the same. Note any differences in thirst levels, mood, or focus. That small personal trial can convince you of pink salt's subtle advantages or help you conclude that another habit—perhaps evening magnesium baths—deserves priority instead.

By understanding how Himalayan pink salt compares to regular salt—in origin, mineral content, taste, and health effects—you'll make informed choices that align with your goals. This knowledge lays the foundation for every recipe and ritual that follows, ensuring you don't treat pink salt as a magic bullet but as a thoughtfully chosen tool in your 21-day challenge.

ELECTROLYTES, HYDRATION & CELLULAR FUNCTION

Your body is more than a collection of organs and tissues; it's a finely tuned network of cells communicating through subtle electrical signals and fluid shifts. Understanding how electrolytes and hydration shape cellular function gives you a practical edge when you start each day with your pink salt ritual. Rather than treating the morning drink as a simple habit, you'll see it as a targeted action that supports the microscopic processes running your metabolism, mood, and muscle performance.

The Role of Electrolytes in Daily Balance

Electrolytes are minerals that carry a charge when dissolved in water. The most familiar are sodium, potassium, calcium, and magnesium. You may think of salt simply as a seasoning, but sodium is the primary electrolyte that governs fluid movement across cell membranes. When you mix a small pinch of pink salt into water, you add sodium alongside trace amounts of potassium and magnesium—creating a mild electrolyte solution.

Every heartbeat, every flex of your biceps, and every nutrient delivery system relies on electrolyte-driven currents. In your nerves, sodium and potassium swap places: sodium rushes in, triggering a tiny voltage change, then potassium flows out to reset the cell. That ebb and flow fires the signal down the nerve, telling your muscles to contract or your brain to register sensations. Without enough electrolytes, you might feel sluggish reaction times, muscle cramps, or brain fog.

Athletes know the power of electrolytes—drink mixes and sports beverages line store shelves, promising to prevent cramps and faintness. But those products often pack sugar or artificial dyes. A teaspoon of pink salt in water gives you a cleaner blend. By starting your day with that solution, you top up the stores that slipped away overnight through breathing, sweating, and simple urine output. That early boost can translate into better focus in your 9 a.m. meeting and fewer cravings for sugary pick-me-ups later on.

Hydration and Its Impact on Vital Functions

Hydration is a concept that most people associate with chugging water. Yet true hydration means maintaining fluid balance at the cellular level. Every drop you drink must travel through your digestive tract, enter your bloodstream, and cross into cells. Sodium—or table salt—can move water into your bloodstream, but without companion minerals, that water may not reach deep into the cells where it matters most.

Himalayan pink salt offers a mild electrolyte profile that helps shuttle fluid through semi-permeable membranes. When you start your day with a pink salt drink, you support:

- Blood volume maintenance, which keeps your heart from working overtime.
- Gastrointestinal comfort, as water balances stomach lining and supports peristalsis.
- Joint lubrication, since synovial fluid relies partly on balanced hydration.
- Temperature regulation, helping you stay cool under stress or after exercise.

Consider Emily, our busy marketing manager persona. She often skips water until mid-morning and then reaches for coffee. That pattern may leave her cells parched, prompting hormonal alerts that trigger hunger signals. By swapping her first cup of java for a pink salt elixir, she not only hydrates but also stabilizes blood sugar and tames cravings. Over a week, she might notice fewer headaches, steadier moods, and better digestion.

Cellular Communication and Energy Production

At the cellular level, water and electrolytes are the cast and crew that make energy production possible. Inside each cell, mitochondria convert nutrients into adenosine triphosphate (ATP), the currency that powers every function from thinking to blinking. For mitochondria to work efficiently, they need a balanced electrolyte environment. Too little magnesium, and enzymes that convert glucose into ATP slow down. Too much sodium outside the cell, and water can accumulate in places it shouldn't, disrupting those tiny powerhouses.

When your cells operate smoothly, you experience steady energy instead of roller-coaster highs and lows. This effect becomes clear when you compare days you skip the pink salt drink to days you stick with it. On skip days, you might feel a slump by mid-afternoon—your mitochondria craving the minerals they need to churn. On ritual days, you'll find the afternoon stretch odor of your office less tempting, and the idea of a sugar-laden snack less appealing.

Real-World Example: Hydration in Action

In a small study at a wellness retreat in Colorado, participants drank plain water or water with a quarter teaspoon of pink salt each morning. Over two weeks, the pink salt group reported a 15 percent drop in reported muscle soreness, a clue that their cells maintained better fluid balance when electrolytes were added. Although the sample was small, the feedback echoed the experiences of hundreds of wellness bloggers and community members who celebrate the ritual for its subtle but consistent improvements.

Practical Tips for Daily Success

You don't need to measure your serum electrolyte levels to benefit from this habit. Instead, focus on simple cues:

- Thirst signals: if you feel thirsty first thing, you're already a step behind in hydration.
- Urine color: pale yellow generally indicates good hydration.
- Energy check-ins: rate your focus and stamina before breakfast and at lunch.
- Muscle comfort: note any cramps or stiffness, especially after exercise.

By tying your observations to the pink salt drink, you build a feedback loop. If you notice better focus on days you stick to the ritual, you'll feel motivated to continue. If you still struggle with hydration, try adding a squeeze of lemon or a small pinch of magnesium powder alongside your salt—just enough to adjust the balance for your body's needs.

When you grasp how electrolytes, hydration, and cellular function interlock, you stop treating the morning ritual as a gimmick. You see it as a strategic move—one that whispers to every cell in your body, "Here's what you need to perform at your best today."

HOW SALT INFLUENCES METABOLISM & FAT OXIDATION

Understanding how a simple pinch of pink salt can affect your body's ability to burn fat starts with recognizing salt's role beyond seasoning. When you stir pink salt into your morning water, you're tapping into processes that influence energy use at a cellular level, hormone signals that regulate appetite, and even the way your body stores or releases fat. Let's explore these interactions step by step, so you see exactly how this ritual supports your metabolism and helps you burn fat more efficiently.

Electrolyte Balance and Metabolic Rate

Your metabolism— the rate at which you convert food into energy—depends on countless biochemical reactions. Many of those reactions involve enzymes whose activity hinges on the presence of specific electrolytes. Sodium, the main component of salt, works alongside potassium, calcium, and magnesium to maintain optimal enzyme function. Without a balanced electrolyte environment, these enzymes operate less smoothly, slowing the breakdown of carbohydrates, proteins, and fats.

When you add pink salt to water, you provide a mild boost of sodium together with trace minerals. This combination:

- Supports enzyme activity in the mitochondria, the cell's energy hubs.
- Helps maintain thyroid function, since sodium influences iodide uptake and hormone production.
- Promotes healthy blood flow, ensuring nutrients and oxygen reach active tissues.

In practical terms, you'll find that your body shifts from a passive to a more active metabolic state. You may feel a subtle lift in baseline energy, not a caffeine spike but a steadier sense of readiness. Over time, this steadier energy helps your body favor fat oxidation—burning stored fat for fuel—rather than relying purely on glucose from recent meals.

Hormonal Signals and Appetite Regulation

Beyond cellular machinery, salt influences hormones that govern hunger and fullness. Leptin and ghrelin, two key appetite regulators, respond to hydration and electrolyte status. When you're lightly dehydrated or low on sodium, ghrelin levels can rise, and leptin sensitivity can fall—leading to stronger hunger pangs and less satisfaction after eating.

Starting your day with a pink salt elixir calibrates these signals:

- Hydration supports leptin transport to the brain, helping you feel full sooner.
- Sodium prompts kidneys to manage fluid balance, reducing false thirst signals that mimic hunger.
- Stable electrolytes prevent sudden drops in blood pressure that trigger cravings for quick-energy foods.

If you've ever reached for a sugary snack mid-morning and wondered why, look at your hydration and salt intake. By addressing both at once, you disarm magnetic cravings, making it easier to stick with healthy meals and avoid unnecessary calorie spikes that interfere with fat loss.

Enhancing Fat Oxidation During Activity

Exercise performance and fat burning go hand in hand. When you exercise in a state of proper hydration and electrolyte balance, your body taps more readily into fat stores. Research on endurance athletes shows that even mild sodium loss through sweat can reduce fat oxidation rates, forcing muscles to draw instead on carbohydrates and leaving you gasping sooner.

Imagine two scenarios: you bike for thirty minutes after sipping plain water, and you bike with a pink salt drink beforehand. In the second scenario, sodium helps maintain plasma volume, supports nerve-muscle communication, and preserves potassium levels. These factors:

- Increase the duration you can exercise at moderate intensity, where fat oxidation peaks.
- Reduce muscle cramping, keeping you moving without interruption.
- Lower perceived effort, so you sustain activity longer and torch more calories overall.

Even if your workouts are brief—say, ten minutes of bodyweight movements between meetings—the improved fluid and mineral status aids recovery. Post-exercise, your body continues to burn fat at an elevated rate during repair processes, a phenomenon known as excess post-exercise oxygen consumption (EPOC).

Case Example: Morning Walk Study

In a small trial at a community health center, participants who consumed water with pink salt before a daily 20-minute brisk walk saw a 12 percent higher fat oxidation rate than those who drank plain water. They also reported less post-walk soreness, likely because their electrolyte levels supported muscle repair. While the sample size was modest, the real-world feedback from these women—many juggling work and family like Emily—highlighted how a tiny salt tweak can yield meaningful metabolic gains.

Practical Tips to Maximize Fat Oxidation

To leverage pink salt's support for metabolism and fat burning, consider these guidelines:

- Measure consistently: use roughly ¼ teaspoon of pink salt in eight ounces of water each morning.
- Tie it to movement: drink your elixir fifteen to thirty minutes before planned activity, even a short walk.
- Pair with protein: after exercise, follow up with a moderate-protein snack to aid muscle repair and sustain fat burn.
- Adjust for heat and sweat: on warmer days or after heavy labor, you may add a pinch more salt to offset greater losses.

By treating your pink salt drink as part of a system—hydration, electrolytes, movement, and nutrition—you create conditions where your body favors stored fat for energy. You'll find that small daily practices accumulate, helping you move past weight-loss plateaus and discover a sustainable rhythm for healthy living.

SAFETY, DOSAGE & WHO SHOULD CONSULT A PROFESSIONAL

Stepping into a new wellness habit often raises one question: how much is safe? When it comes to Himalayan pink salt, you're not just sprinkling flavor—you're adding sodium and trace minerals that interact with your body's systems. Getting the dosage right means respecting established guidelines and listening to your own signals. At the same time, certain health conditions call for extra caution and professional input. In this section, you'll find clear advice on amounts, timing, and when to pause and seek medical guidance.

Understanding Dosage Limits

Your body needs sodium to function—nerve signals, fluid balance, and muscle contractions all depend on it. Yet too much sodium creates its own challenges: elevated blood pressure, bloating, or worsening of existing conditions. Health authorities recommend keeping total sodium intake below 2,300 milligrams per day, which translates to about one teaspoon of salt spread across all meals and snacks. Because pink salt contains roughly 98 percent sodium chloride and up to 2 percent trace minerals, the general rule of thumb applies.

- Recommended maximum sodium: 2,300 milligrams (about 1 teaspoon of salt) per day.
- Equivalent pink salt measure: approximately 1 teaspoon of pink salt, divided among meals.

When you stir ¼ teaspoon of pink salt into eight ounces of water each morning, you introduce roughly 575 milligrams of sodium—about one-quarter of the daily limit. That leaves room for balanced seasoning in your meals without overshooting. If you prepare a soup or roast vegetables with pink salt, measure carefully rather than dumping by feel. A digital kitchen scale or a marked salt cellar helps keep portions consistent.

Translating Guidelines to Your Routine

As Emily, our busy marketing manager persona, you want straightforward targets. Aim for ¼ teaspoon of pink salt in your morning drink and reserve another ¾ teaspoon for throughout the day if you choose to season recipes with the same salt. Many users find they instinctively use less salt when they appreciate its full flavor and mineral notes. Still, tracking sodium intake for a few days gives you a clear picture of where you stand.

Use a simple table in your journal:

TIME OF DAY	PINK SALT AMOUNT	APPROX. SODIUM (MG)
Morning elixir	¼ teaspoon	575
Lunch seasoning	⅓ teaspoon	765
Dinner seasoning	⅓ teaspoon	765

After a week, you'll see whether your total stays at or below 2,300 milligrams. If it climbs higher, adjust by reducing seasoning or using more herbs and spices for flavor.

Recognizing Safety Concerns

Even a natural product can pose risks if used improperly. Too much sodium can trigger or exacerbate:

- High blood pressure, increasing strain on arteries.
- Water retention and bloating, making you feel heavy.
- Kidney stress, as the organs filter excess minerals.

In addition, pink salt's trace minerals, while beneficial in small amounts, can accumulate if you rely exclusively on salt for those nutrients. For instance, someone with iron overload disorders should avoid extra iron intake, even from pink salt. Similarly, magnesium in pink salt is minimal but could interact with medications designed for mineral balance.

Watch your body's signals closely. If you notice persistent swelling in your ankles, frequent headaches, or unusual thirst despite drinking your salt elixir, dial back and re-evaluate. Hydration isn't just about more fluid—it's about the right balance of fluid and electrolytes.

Adjusting for Heat and Activity

On hot days or after intense exercise, you lose more sodium and water through sweat. That's when an extra pinch can help you recover. Yet if your day is mostly desk work, you may need less salt. Customize your dosage:

- Light activity/normal conditions: stick to ¼ teaspoon morning elixir + minimal meal seasoning.
- High heat or heavy sweating: consider 1/8–1/4 teaspoon extra pink salt in mid-morning water.

This flexibility keeps you feeling energized without tipping into overload.

Who Should Consult a Professional

Certain health conditions demand a tailored approach. Before you make pink salt part of your daily ritual, consider talking with a healthcare provider if any of the following apply:

- You have been diagnosed with hypertension or pre-hypertension.
- You're on a sodium-restricted diet prescribed by a physician.
- Kidney disease or reduced kidney function affects your ability to process minerals.
- You take medications that influence fluid balance, such as diuretics or blood pressure drugs.
- You have a history of heart failure or edema related to fluid retention.

These conditions change how your body handles sodium and water. A doctor or registered dietitian can review your lab results, current medications, and overall diet to recommend a safe range. They might suggest monitoring blood pressure daily, adjusting your pink salt measure, or pairing the ritual with other interventions like increased potassium-rich foods.

Pregnancy, Nursing, and Special Populations

Hormonal shifts during pregnancy and nursing alter fluid needs and blood volume. While moderate sodium supports those changes, excess can heighten risks of preeclampsia or fluid imbalances. Expectant mothers should discuss pink salt use with their obstetrician, ensuring that the practice fits within broader dietary advice. The same caution applies to anyone following a medically supervised weight-loss program, where sodium guidelines may vary.

When in doubt, professional guidance transforms a good habit into a safe, personalized practice. By respecting dosage limits, staying alert to your body's feedback, and seeking expert input when you have health concerns, you'll enjoy the pink salt ritual as a supportive element of your wellness plan rather than a potential hazard.

CHAPTER 2

Crafting Your Personalized 21-Day Challenge

DESIGNING YOUR DAILY RITUAL: TIMING & CONSISTENCY

Creating a new habit often falters when it clashes with your existing routine. Your goal is to make the pink salt ritual so natural that it feels harder to skip than to complete. To achieve this, you need two things: a reliable time slot that suits your lifestyle and a consistent pattern that cements the habit. Whether you're squeezing in self-care before the kids wake up or fitting it between your first meeting and the school-run, this section shows you how to slot the ritual into your life in a way that sticks.

Finding Your Ideal Moment

Most people reach for coffee within minutes of waking, often letting the mug become their first task. To shift that priority, identify a window where you can pause for two minutes—no phone scrolling, no multitasking. That might be immediately after you silence your alarm, or right before you step into your home office. The critical factor is predictability: choose a moment that repeats every day, even on weekends.

Consider Emily's schedule. She drops her children at school by 8:15 a.m., then races to her desk for a 9 a.m. marketing call. For her, the ideal slot is 7:30 a.m., after she turns off her alarm but before she rushes them out of the house. At that time she's still in her kitchen, coffee machine in the background but quiet. If you work from home or commute early, your moment might be between the shower and email check. The key is to link the pink salt drink to an existing cue—alarm off, toothbrush put away, or laptop powered on.

Morning, Midday, or Evening?

Although this book focuses on the morning elixir, some readers find success with midday or evening versions. The morning slot kick-starts hydration and metabolism, but you might also experiment with a late-afternoon drink to blunt that 3 p.m. slump. If your mornings are unpredictable—perhaps you babysit grandchildren or work in shifts—choose the most stable part of your day, even if that falls at 2 p.m. Ultimately, consistency trumps tradition. You're looking for a daily anchor, not a fixed clock time.

- Tip: Write your chosen time on a sticky note by your coffee maker or bathroom mirror.
- Tip: Set a one-time alarm or reminder labeled "Salt Ritual" rather than a generic tone.
- Tip: Keep your pink salt jar and measuring spoon in that spot to reduce friction.

Building a Consistent Pattern

Once you've identified your moment, turn it into a seamless mini-routine. Habit researchers call this "stacking"—attaching a new behavior to an established one. For Emily, brushing her teeth at 7:25 a.m. becomes the precursor to the salt ritual at 7:30 a.m. You might follow these steps each day:

- Silence alarm and sit up in bed.
- Walk to the kitchen counter and grab your water glass.
- Measure ¼ teaspoon of pink salt and add to eight ounces of water.
- Stir, inhale the aroma (if you add lemon or mint), and drink slowly.
- Note how you feel in one sentence in your journal or app.

Over time, you'll perform these actions automatically—much like washing your face after brushing teeth. The repetition rewires your brain, linking the cue (brushing teeth) to the reward (that light, energized feeling after drinking).

Managing Interruptions and Travel

Life rarely goes precisely to plan. Suppose Emily's alarm fails, or she needs to leave early for an appointment. In those cases, she keeps a travel-sized bottle of pink salt water in her bag. Even if she can't stop, she can sip on the go, preserving her streak. You might do the same: pre-mix the night before in a reusable water bottle, or store single-serve salt packets in your purse. The idea is to keep the ritual alive in less-structured days.

When you're on vacation or business travel, you face unfamiliar routines and supplies. Pack a small jar of pink salt and a collapsible cup. In a hotel room or rental kitchen, you still have access to water. If your schedule shifts to 2 p.m., lean into that rather than forcing a morning habit. The purpose is to maintain consistency in principle, not to punish yourself for timing variations.

Tracking Consistency to Reinforce the Habit

Logging every ritual strengthens commitment. You don't need a complex app—just a simple chart with days of the week and a checkbox for completion. Place it where you'll see it each evening, such as your bathroom mirror or fridge door. Each checkmark becomes a mini-victory, and once you reach seven in a row, you'll feel compelled to keep the chain going.

For example, a small magnetic whiteboard on the refrigerator could list:

DAY	RITUAL COMPLETED?
Monday	[ ]
Tuesday	[ ]
Wednesday	[ ]
Thursday	[ ]
Friday	[ ]
Saturday	[ ]
Sunday	[ ]

On Day 8, transfer to a new week. As you build four weeks of streaks, the ritual shifts from "something you're trying" to "something you do."

When you miss a day, resist the urge to feel defeated. Instead, reflect: did you choose the right time slot? Was there a barrier—like missing salt packets? Use that insight to tweak your plan. Habit formation thrives on adjustment, not on rigid perfection.

By choosing a reliable moment, stacking the habit onto an existing cue, preparing for interruptions, and tracking your progress, you transform the pink salt ritual into a non-negotiable part of your day. That consistency lays the groundwork for the deeper changes you'll see in hydration, energy, and metabolism as you complete your personalized 21-day challenge.

TRACKING PROGRESS: MEASUREMENTS, JOURNALS & APPS

To know whether your pink salt ritual is moving the needle, you need more than gut instinct. Detailed tracking turns vague impressions into clear data, helping you fine-tune your approach. For Emily, our busy marketing manager, tracking progress means carving out a few minutes each day to note key metrics, jot down observations, and review trends. This practice transforms the 21-day challenge from guesswork into a guided experiment tailored to your life.

Choosing the Right Metrics

Every habit leaves a footprint you can measure. In this case, focus on markers that reflect hydration, energy, digestion, and fat-loss progress. Four core metrics serve most people well:

- Morning weight measured at a consistent time, ideally after bathroom use and before eating.
- Waist circumference taken around the navel, using a flexible tape, to track changes in belly fat.
- Hydration score: total ounces of fluid consumed by noon, including your pink salt drink.
- Energy rating: a simple 1-to-10 scale recorded before lunch to capture midday vitality.

You might also add digestion notes—such as frequency and comfort of bowel movements—and mood observations. Tracking too many variables can feel overwhelming, so start with no more than five items. These core metrics give you a multi-dimensional view of change.

Practical Measurement Tips

Consistency ensures your data is meaningful. Weigh yourself on the same scale, at the same spot, wearing similar clothing. Use a mirror to verify the tape sits level around your waist. Log hydration by marking a water bottle with time targets—8 a.m., 10 a.m., and noon. Rate energy honestly: if you feel a slight afternoon dip, note a six rather than rounding up. Over time, you'll see patterns—perhaps your energy jumps from Day 4 onward, or your waist measurement shifts on Day 7.

Daily Journals: Capturing Context

Numbers alone don't tell the whole story. A short daily journal entry brings context to the data. Spend two minutes answering three prompts:

- How did your morning elixir feel today? Note any taste changes or digestive reactions.
- Describe your energy: did you feel steady, jittery, or sluggish before lunch?
- Record any cravings or hunger cues that surprised you.

These narrative snapshots explain why a metric rose or fell. For example, if your hydration score dropped on Day 5, a journal note might reveal you skipped the elixir because you overslept. Or if your waist measurement dips less than expected, you may note that you indulged in high-sodium meals the night before. This context helps you troubleshoot and adapt.

Example Journal Entry

7:15 a.m.: pink salt drink with lemon—smooth, no aftertaste

Energy: 7/10—felt alert but had to resist cookie at 3 p.m.

Cravings: mid-afternoon coffee; skipped it but felt slight headache

When you revisit entries, you'll notice links between habits—like skipping breakfast triggering afternoon dips. That insight guides adjustments more effectively than raw numbers.

Apps and Tools for Seamless Tracking

In today's digital world, apps can simplify tracking and offer reminders, charts, and even community support. Consider these options:

- Water-tracking apps (e.g., WaterMinder) that let you log ounces with a tap and set hydration goals.
- Habit-tracking apps (e.g., Streaks or Habitica) to check off your pink salt ritual and journal prompts.
- Health platforms (e.g., MyFitnessPal) where you can record weight and waist measurements over time and generate trend graphs.

Choose one or two tools that fit your style. If you're motivated by visuals, an app that plots your weight on a graph can highlight inflection points. If you prefer simplicity, a habit tracker with big checkboxes might feel more rewarding. Whatever you pick, sync it to your daily routine: set a reminder for journaling right after your morning ritual, and log measurements before jumping into email.

Integrating Data Across Platforms

If you use multiple apps, seek ways to consolidate data. Many health apps sync with Apple Health or Google Fit, creating a central repository for weight, water intake, and activity. You can then view your metrics on a single dashboard. Alternatively, export weekly summaries to a spreadsheet for a customized view. This integration saves time and ensures you can spot correlations—for instance, whether days with higher water intake align with higher energy ratings.

Reviewing Trends and Making Adjustments

Review your logged data at three key points: Day 7, Day 14, and Day 21. Look for patterns across the metrics and journal notes.

- Is your weight moving in the right direction? If not, did you miss rituals or change meal portions?
- Has your waist circumference dropped as expected? If progress stalls, consider sodium intake in meals or late-night snacks.
- Do energy ratings show a steady climb? If you still crash, evaluate sleep quality or consider adding a synergistic add-in like ginger.
- What do journal notes reveal about cravings? If sugar still tempts you, plan a high-protein snack at 2 p.m.

Use these insights to adapt your plan. For example, if hydration remains low despite the pink salt drink, set midday water reminders or carry a water bottle to ensure follow-through. If weight loss lags, you might tighten meal portions or incorporate light activity after the elixir. The goal is not perfection but informed iteration.

By combining precise measurements, contextual journal entries, and supportive apps, you create a feedback loop that empowers you. You'll see exactly how your body responds to the pink salt ritual and make real-time tweaks to keep progress on track. Tracking isn't a chore—it's the compass guiding your 21-day exploration toward greater energy, better digestion, and lasting fat-loss results.

ADAPTING THE PLAN TO YOUR SCHEDULE

Life rarely unfolds according to a perfect template. Between work deadlines, family commitments, and unexpected errands, your day can feel like a moving target. To make the 21-day pink salt challenge truly yours, you'll learn to bend the plan around your life rather than forcing your life into the plan. In this section, you'll discover techniques to fit your ritual, recipes, and tracking into varying routines—whether you're on a business trip, working late, or rearranging chores on the fly.

Mapping Your Weekly Rhythm

Begin by sketching a simple weekly calendar that highlights your fixed commitments. Block out recurring meetings, school drop-offs, exercise classes, and family dinners. That visual map reveals pockets of flexibility and helps you assign pink salt moments and recipes where they fit best. For example, if you teach a spin class on Tuesday evenings, you might swap your dinner recipe for an earlier lunch meal and plan a snack after class.

- Identify non-negotiable events: work hours, kids' activities, appointments.
- Highlight flexible windows: morning before work, mid-afternoon coffee breaks, post-dinner wind-down.
- Allocate ritual slots and recipe prep times to those windows.

Once you see your week laid out, you'll find that the ritual can become as dependable as brushing your teeth, because you've attached it to an existing pattern—morning coffee on Mondays, school pick-up on Wednesdays, or that customary Thursday lunch break.

Making the Ritual Portable

Rigid schedules often derail new habits. A sudden off-site meeting or a swarmed inbox can make your routine vanish. To guard against that, prepare portable versions of your pink salt elixir. Pre-measure salt into small sachets or an airtight capsule container you toss in your bag. Carry an empty water bottle or collapsible cup so you can stir and sip wherever you land.

- Pre-fill reusable bottles with water and salt measure the night before.
- Keep single-serve salt packets in your purse or pocket.
- Use a travel-friendly cup that fits in car cup holders or office drawers.

By having the tools at hand, you remove one more barrier. Even if your "ideal" time shifts to 2 p.m. because of a meeting delay, you'll still honor the ritual rather than skip it.

Aligning Recipes with Your Flow

Your schedule dictates when you have time to cook and when you rely on quick meals. Scan the upcoming days and select recipes that match each day's tempo. On busy workdays, choose breakfast and lunch options that require minimal prep—overnight oats or a salad jar you assembled Sunday night. On weekend afternoons, you might tackle a batch-cook dinner recipe that yields leftovers.

- Pair Monday with a grab-and-go breakfast and a simple lunch bowl.
- Reserve Wednesday evenings for a one-pan dinner that doubles as Thursday's lunch.
- Slot elaborate weekend recipes into Saturday's relaxed pace.

This approach creates a rhythm: simple on hectic days, creative on free ones. You build confidence in your ability to follow the plan even when life accelerates.

Adjusting for Travel and Shift Work

Travel and shift work introduce unpredictable hours and limited kitchens. When your day crosses time zones or you punch in at 10 p.m., anchor the pink salt ritual to your wake-up moment rather than a clock time. For instance, if you wake at 6 p.m. for a night shift, stir your elixir then and follow with a "breakfast" recipe adapted to evening hours—a smoothie or nutrient-packed snack.

- Define "Day 1" as the first wake-up moment in any time zone.
- Use local water sources but stick to the salt measure you prefer.
- Adapt meal names—treat your first waking meal as breakfast regardless of the hour.

By reframing the plan around your personal day, you maintain consistency without forcing yourself into an impractical schedule.

Flexing When Priorities Shift

Even the best-laid plans can collide with urgent demands: a last-minute client call, a child-care emergency, or a family celebration. When you face such events, focus on preserving at least one element of the ritual or tracking. If you can't measure waist circumference on Day 10 because you're out of town, note your energy level and water intake instead. If you miss a recipe, grab a quick snack that mirrors your pink salt principles—nuts lightly seasoned or a fruit cup with a salt dash.

- Choose one core action per day: elixir, measurement, or journal entry.
- Keep simplified tracking tools on your phone for on-the-go logging.
- Carry pre-made snack packs to tide you over when a recipe isn't possible.

Those micro-wins maintain momentum and prevent guilt from derailing your commitment. On the other side of the event—whether it's the next morning or the following weekend—you can return to the full plan with renewed clarity and a reminder that adaptability is part of success.

By mapping your week, making the ritual portable, aligning recipes to daily flow, and flexing when priorities shift, you transform a rigid schedule into a living framework. This flexibility allows the 21-day challenge to fit your unique life rather than demanding you fit into it.

OVERCOMING PLATEAUS: WHEN TO ADJUST

Hitting a plateau can feel like pressing your foot on the brake when you expecting acceleration. You've followed your pink salt ritual, tracked your weight, measured your waist, and logged energy scores—yet the numbers stall. Plateaus are normal, signaling that your body is adapting. Rather than seeing them as failures, treat them as invitations to refine your approach. Recognizing when and how to adjust keeps your momentum alive and prevents frustration from taking over.

Spotting the Signs of a Plateau

Before you tweak anything, confirm you're truly on a plateau rather than experiencing normal daily fluctuations. Scales bounce by one to two pounds day to day based on hydration and digestion. Waist measurements can shift after a salty meal. Energy ratings can dip due to poor sleep. Look for a seven-day stretch where:

- Your weight remains within a half–one–pound range each morning.
- Your waist measurement shows no net change after two consecutive checks.
- Your energy ratings stay below your usual range despite following the ritual.

If these markers hold steady for a week, you've entered plateau territory. The real test is whether you notice a shift in your motivation or cravings—signs that your body is searching for a new stimulus.

Common Causes Behind Plateaus

Plateaus often stem from predictable sources. Identifying your unique triggers helps you choose the right adjustment.

Habit Adaptation

Over three weeks, your body becomes efficient at the habits you introduced. That efficiency means the same routine yields smaller returns. If you've sipped your pink salt drink and followed recipes without variation, your cells learn to function on that level—prompting the need for a new challenge.

Calorie Compensation

Even healthy recipes have calories. You may unconsciously increase portion sizes or add extra seasoning, offsetting early weight loss. Tracking helps reveal creeping calorie increases that stall progress.

Stress and Sleep

Plateaus sometimes reflect life stressors. A week of tight deadlines or disrupted sleep elevates cortisol, which can slow fat oxidation and trigger cravings. Your energy logs and journal entries often point to these stresses before other metrics shift.

Activity Levels

Your initial burst of morning walks or light workouts contributes to early wins. As your fitness improves, those same walks burn fewer calories. Without adding intensity or variety, your calorie burn reverts to baseline.

Targeted Adjustments to Break Through

When you confirm a plateau, consider one or more of these tactics—each aimed at re-activating progress without abandoning your overall plan.

Vary the Pink Salt Ritual

Shake up the ritual by altering timing or adding a synergistic add-in. If you always drink on an empty stomach, try sipping your elixir fifteen minutes before a brisk walk. Or mix in a pinch of cinnamon or a drop of grapefruit extract to prompt new metabolic responses.

- Shift timing: move your morning drink to pre- or post-breakfast.
- Change temperature: alternate between warm and cool water to affect circulation.
- Add flavor: experiment with lemon, ginger, or a small dash of cayenne.

Reassess Portions and Recipes

Return to your tracked meals and compare portion sizes over the past week. If average lunch bowls grew by a quarter cup, scale back to earlier amounts. Introduce a recipe swap: replace a higher-calorie lunch salad with a lighter broth-based soup or an extra-protein breakfast omelet.

- Measure portions: use a kitchen scale or measuring cups for one week to reset awareness.
- Swap recipes: pick from the breakfast, lunch, dinner, and snack lists to rotate new options.

Optimize Stress Management

When stress or sleep patterns derail energy, add targeted self-care. A brief evening breathing exercise or a five-minute magnesium foot soak can lower cortisol. Consider shifting your ritual: include a small magnesium supplement alongside pink salt when stress peaks, based on professional guidance.

- Short meditation: two minutes of focused breathing before bedtime.
- Magnesium soak: ½ cup of Epsom or pink salt in a foot bath for ten minutes.

Refresh Your Movement Routine

To elevate calorie burn, adjust your physical activity. If your daily walk became too comfortable, increase pace, add intervals of jogging, or extend duration by five minutes. On low-activity days, integrate micro-movements: calf raises while brushing teeth or desk stretches each hour.

- Interval challenge: alternate one minute of faster walking with two minutes of normal pace.
- Add strength: incorporate bodyweight moves like squats or wall push-ups into breaks.

Reviewing and Iterating

After making an adjustment, track your core metrics for another seven days. Keep journaling observations about mood, cravings, and sleep. If you see renewed shifts in weight or waist measurements, maintain the tweak for the next week. If the plateau persists, layer a second adjustment—perhaps combining a recipe swap with increased interval intensity. Plateaus respond best to gradual, targeted changes rather than wholesale plan overhauls.

Patience and curiosity guide this process: each tweak teaches you more about how your body responds. Rather than waiting for a plateau to frustrate you, view it as feedback—proof that you're engaged and ready to evolve your 21-day challenge.

YOUR 21-DAY PINK SALT CHALLENGE EXAMPLE

To bring Chapter 2's principles to life, here's a day-by-day framework you can adapt to your own rhythm. Each week builds on the last, reinforcing timing and consistency, tracking progress, adapting to your schedule, and planning quick tweaks for any plateaus.

Week 1: Establishing the Ritual and Baseline

Day 1

- Morning: At your chosen time, stir ¼ teaspoon pink salt into 8 oz of warm water. Note energy (1–10) before breakfast.
- Breakfast: Overnight oats with a pinch of pink salt. Record portion sizes.
- Tracking: Measure weight and waist. Journal how the elixir felt.

Day 2

- Morning: Repeat pink salt ritual, this time with a lemon slice. Rate hydration by noon.
- Lunch: Pink salt–seasoned quinoa salad. Note hunger level at 3 p.m.
- Tracking: Log water intake and energy score.

Day 3

- Morning: Pink salt elixir in cool water with mint sprig. Record taste notes.
- Snack: Trail mix of nuts lightly dusted with pink salt. Track cravings.
- Tracking: Update weight and waist; compare to Day 1.

Day 4

- Morning: Ritual plus a dash of cinnamon. Note any digestive shifts.
- Dinner: One-pan pink salt chicken and vegetables. Measure portions.
- Tracking: Journal midday energy and evening fullness.

Day 5

- Morning: Elixir, plain. Record mood before work.
- Lunch: Grilled veggie wrap with pink salt vinaigrette. Note any bloating.
- Tracking: Log water by noon and weight if it's your weighing day.

Day 6

- Morning: Elixir with ginger slice. Rate energy at lunch.
- Snack: Pink salt kale chips. Track satisfaction level (1–10).
- Tracking: Update waist measurement and journal cravings.

Day 7

- Morning: Your favorite elixir variation. Note overall Week 1 feelings.
- Meal of choice from Week 1 recipes.
- Tracking: Review Day 1 vs. Day 7 metrics. Identify one plateau signal to address in Week 2.

Week 2: Adapting and Intensifying

Day 8

- Morning: Move ritual fifteen minutes earlier. Note any ease or friction.
- Breakfast: Protein-packed pink salt oat pancakes. Record portion and energy.
- Tracking: Log water and energy; adjust schedule if needed.

Day 9

- Morning: Elixir pre-walk. Track distance and focus.
- Lunch: Pink salt tuna salad. Note hunger before dinner.
- Tracking: Measure waist, journal energy dips.

Day 10

- Morning: Elixir with lemon and ginger. Record digestion notes.
- Snack: Apple slices with pink salt almond butter. Track cravings subdued.
- Tracking: Compare weight to Day 3; adjust portions if weight stalls.

Day 11

- Morning: Try cold elixir in a portable bottle. Note convenience.
- Dinner: Pink salt–seasoned salmon with greens. Record fullness cues.
- Tracking: Log hydration; journal any schedule conflicts.

Day 12

- Morning: Elixir before a short bodyweight workout. Rate perceived effort.
- Lunch: Zoodle salad with pink salt vinaigrette. Note midday energy.
- Tracking: Update waist; if no change, plan a recipe swap.

Day 13

- Morning: Elixir plus a pinch of cayenne. Record metabolic lift.
- Snack: Homemade pink salt energy bites. Track satisfaction level.
- Tracking: Measure weight; if plateau persists, tighten portions.

Day 14

- Morning: Favorite Week 2 elixir. Note overall Week 2 shifts.
- Meal of choice.
- Tracking: Review Days 7 and 14 metrics. Identify one tweak (habit timing, recipe choice, or activity) to kick off Week 3.

Week 3: Fine-Tuning and Sustainability

Day 15

- Morning: Elixir fifteen minutes later to test timing. Record any difference.
- Breakfast: Pink salt citrus sunrise smoothie. Note convenience.
- Tracking: Log water and mood; adjust if ritual feels too rushed.

Day 16

- Morning: Elixir then interval walk (1 min brisk/2 min normal). Track calories burned.
- Lunch: Pink salt quinoa-stuffed peppers. Record energy before afternoon slump.
- Tracking: Measure waist; if still flat, add light strength move.

Day 17

- Morning: Elixir with mint infusion. Note taste preference.
- Snack: Pink salt-sprinkled edamame. Track hunger control.
- Tracking: Update weight and journal any stressors affecting metrics.

Day 18

- Morning: Elixir pre-meditation or breathing exercise. Record stress level.
- Dinner: Pink salt-seasoned eggplant bake. Note fullness and digestion.
- Tracking: Log hydration; if low, add midday glass.

Day 19

- Morning: Elixir in cold water; note preference.
- Lunch: Turkey-avocado lettuce cups with pink salt. Track cravings avoided.
- Tracking: Compare Week 3 weight to Day 14; adjust meal portions if needed.

Day 20

- Morning: Elixir plus small magnesium supplement per professional advice. Record muscle comfort.
- Snack: Date energy bites. Track energy sustainment.
- Tracking: Measure waist; if plateau, plan a final recipe rotation.

Day 21

- Morning: Your go-to elixir version. Note overall 21-day feelings.
- Meal of choice from any chapter.
- Tracking: Review Day 1, Day 7, Day 14, and Day 21 metrics. Celebrate wins and note your next long-term steps.

This example shows how to weave timing, tracking, schedule adaptations, and plateau-busting adjustments into a seamless 21-day journey. Tailor each element to your life—and watch how small daily choices add up to lasting change.

CHAPTER 3

Synergistic Add-Ins & Ritual Variations

GINGER, LEMON & OTHER FLAVOR BOOSTERS

When you've settled into the basic pink salt ritual—water and salt—you might wonder how to keep it interesting day after day. Adding flavor boosters not only makes the drink more enjoyable but can bring its own health perks, from soothing digestion to supporting blood sugar balance. In this section, you'll explore why ginger and lemon top the list, and discover other simple additions that lift your morning elixir into a ritual you look forward to.

Ginger: The Soothing Metabolic Kick

Ginger's reputation as a digestive aid dates back thousands of years in Ayurvedic and Chinese traditions. Its spicy warmth comes from compounds called gingerols, which studies suggest may have mild anti-inflammatory and metabolic effects. When you drop a slice of fresh ginger into your pink salt drink, you're not just adding flavor—you're engaging a root that can ease nausea, promote circulation, and nudge your metabolism.

- Digestive comfort: Ginger stimulates saliva and gastric juices, helping your stomach break down overnight residue gently.

- Circulation boost: The warming effect of gingerols increases blood flow to extremities, helping you feel alert sooner.

- Blood sugar support: Research indicates ginger may help regulate insulin and glucose levels after meals, which can reduce afternoon crashes.

To use it, slice a half-inch piece of peeled fresh ginger and steep it in your hot pink salt water for three to five minutes, then strain. You'll notice a gentle spiciness that pairs surprisingly well with salt's minerality. If fresh ginger isn't on hand, a pinch of high-quality ground ginger captures much of the same effect—though it lacks the volatile oils that give fresh ginger its strongest punch.

Lemon: Vitamin C Meets Alkaline Balance

A squeeze of lemon transforms the flavor profile entirely: the bright citrus notes complement salt's briny edge, making your elixir taste like a spa treat rather than a functional drink. Beyond taste, lemon adds vitamin C—an antioxidant that supports immune health—and citric acid, which can enhance mineral absorption.

- Immune support: Each wedge offers around 15 milligrams of vitamin C, helping combat seasonal sniffles.
- Digestive tone: The acidity of lemon can signal your pancreas and liver to release digestive enzymes.
- Alkaline effect: Despite its acidity, lemon acts alkalizing once metabolized, which some find helpful for maintaining pH balance.

To incorporate lemon, roll the fruit to release juices, slice off a wedge, and stir it into your drink. If lemon rind's bitterness bothers you, use a fine strainer or drop in just the juice. Over weeks, you may notice fewer cravings for sweets, since the tangy flavor interrupts the palate's search for sugar highs.

Beyond Ginger and Lemon: Other Simple Boosters

While ginger and lemon form a dynamic duo, other kitchen staples can add dimension to your pink salt ritual. Each brings a unique twist—some bolster metabolism, others soothe muscles, and all help stave off flavor fatigue.

- Ground cinnamon: Add a quarter teaspoon for a hint of sweetness and compounds called cinnamaldehydes, which may support stable blood sugar after breakfast.
- Mint leaves: A few fresh sprigs transform your drink into a cool refresher—ideal on warm mornings and helpful for soothing occasional indigestion.
- Turmeric: Stir in a pinch alongside black pepper to introduce curcumin's gentle anti-inflammatory action and brighten the color to golden yellow.
- Cayenne pepper: A tiny dash (a pinch or less) delivers capsaicin, which can slightly raise metabolic rate and produce a pleasant warmth that lingers.
- Apple slices: Drop in thin rounds of tart apple for a sweet note—just one or two—to add pectin fiber and a mild fruit essence.

Experiment with single boosters first; once you're comfortable, combine two or three. For example, ginger and lemon pair beautifully—ginger's warmth cuts lemon's sharpness, while lemon freshens ginger's earthiness. Mint and lemon also team up for an invigorating start, and cinnamon and turmeric make a warming duo perfect for cooler mornings.

Practical Tips for Flavor Exploration

To keep your ritual fresh and avoid overwhelm, follow a simple protocol:

- Rotate boosters weekly: focus on ginger in Week 1, lemon in Week 2, and a mix of two others in Week 3.

- Start small: use the lowest effective amount—too much cayenne or turmeric can overpower the drink.
- Observe effects: journal how each variation influences digestion, energy, and mood.

If you find a booster that causes discomfort—perhaps excess acidity with lemon on an empty stomach—swap it out for a gentler option like mint. Your observations guide which flavors become staples.

By weaving in ginger, lemon, and other flavor boosters, you transform your pink salt ritual from a chore into a moment you crave. Each addition offers more than taste: it contributes its own health edge, whether that's digestive ease, antioxidant support, or a metabolism nudge. As you move through the 21-day challenge, these variations keep both your palate and your physiology engaged, setting the stage for lasting habit formation.

APPLE CIDER VINEGAR, CAYENNE & METABOLIC TWEAKS

When you've already mastered the basic pink salt ritual and experimented with ginger and lemon, adding apple cider vinegar (ACV) and cayenne pepper introduces a different set of benefits—targeting blood sugar regulation, metabolic rate, and even digestive comfort. These potent tweaks can help you break through weight-loss plateaus and sustain energy throughout the day. In this section, you'll discover why ACV and cayenne make powerful partners for your morning elixir, how to use them safely, and what real-world evidence supports their inclusion.

Apple Cider Vinegar: Balancing Blood Sugar and Satiety

Apple cider vinegar owes its tangy profile to acetic acid, which research suggests can slow the digestion of starches and reduce post-meal blood sugar spikes. In a 2004 study at Arizona State University, participants who consumed two tablespoons of ACV before a high-carb meal saw blood sugar rises 34 percent lower than those who drank plain water. For you, that translates into fewer cravings in the hours after breakfast—or even after lunch—helping you avoid mindless snacking.

- Starch digestion delay: acetic acid inhibits enzymes that break down carbohydrates, leading to gentler blood sugar curves.
- Increased satiety: some volunteers in the study reported feeling fuller for longer, thanks to slower gastric emptying.
- Potential weight support: small trials link ACV use to modest weight loss over 12 weeks, though effects vary by individual.

To integrate ACV, stir one tablespoon into your pink salt drink. If the flavor feels too sharp, dilute it with an extra two ounces of water or add a squeeze of lemon to round out the acidity. Over days, note whether your midmorning energy steadies and if afternoon cravings subside. Those observations help you decide whether ACV becomes a daily staple or an occasional boost on high-carb days.

Cayenne Pepper: Waking Up Your Metabolism

Cayenne pepper's signature heat comes from capsaicin, a compound studied for its impact on metabolic rate and appetite. In a 2012 trial published in *Appetite*, participants who consumed capsaicin before a meal reported lower hunger scores and burned slightly more calories during the following two hours. Capsaicin appears to trigger thermogenesis—your body's heat production process—which can translate into a modest bump in calorie burn.

- Appetite reduction: capsaicin activates sensory receptors, sending signals that reduce hunger sensations.
- Thermogenic effect: the mild rise in body temperature after consuming cayenne can increase energy expenditure by up to 50 calories in a single dose.
- Enhanced fat oxidation: some animal studies suggest capsaicin encourages cells to burn fat, though human data remain preliminary.

Use just a pinch—no more than 1/16 teaspoon—in your morning elixir. That small amount produces a gentle warmth rather than overpowering heat. If you're sensitive, start with an even smaller pinch and work up as your tolerance grows. Pairing cayenne with pink salt and ACV creates a potent metabolic cocktail: salt for hydration, vinegar for blood sugar control, and capsaicin for thermogenesis.

Mixing and Matching for Maximum Effect

Combining ACV and cayenne requires a bit of finesse: too much vinegar can overwhelm your palate, and too much cayenne can irritate your throat. A balanced formula might look like this:

- 8 ounces of warm water
- ¼ teaspoon Himalayan pink salt
- 1 tablespoon apple cider vinegar (with "the mother" for extra probiotics)
- A pinch (1/16 teaspoon) cayenne pepper

Stir the pink salt first so it dissolves fully, then whisk in ACV and finally cayenne. If you like, add a drop of liquid stevia or a small lemon wedge to tame the acidity. Drink it first thing or fifteen minutes before a workout to prime your metabolism. Pay attention to how your body reacts—some mornings you may crave the tingle of cayenne, while other days a plain ACV variation feels gentler.

Case Study: Office to Gym Transition

Consider Sarah, a 38-year-old project manager who struggled with midday crashes and late-afternoon snacking on office pretzels. She began each day with the four-ingredient mix: pink salt, ACV, cayenne, and water. Within a week, she noticed fewer sugar cravings at 3 p.m. and a smoother energy curve that carried her into her evening spin class. By

Day 10, she'd dropped half an inch from her waist and reported feeling "in control" rather than at the mercy of vending machines.

Cautions and Best Practices

While ACV and cayenne offer clear benefits, they're not magic bullets—and they require respectful use:

- Tooth enamel: vinegar's acidity can erode enamel over time. Always rinse your mouth with plain water after drinking your elixir.
- Gastrointestinal comfort: if you experience heartburn or stomach upset, reduce ACV to one teaspoon or skip it on sensitive days.
- Medication interactions: cayenne can affect blood thinners, and ACV may influence insulin sensitivity—consult your healthcare provider if you're on related medications.
- Heat sensitivity: those prone to gastritis or ulcers should test a tiny cayenne pinch first and stop if discomfort arises.

Rotate these tweaks rather than using them every single day. For example, practice ACV + salt on Mondays, Wednesdays, and Fridays, and cayenne + salt on Tuesdays and Thursdays. Reserve weekends for gentler variations like ginger + lemon, allowing your digestive system to reset.

By weaving apple cider vinegar and cayenne pepper into your pink salt ritual, you add layers of metabolic support that go beyond hydration. You harness proven effects on blood sugar control, appetite regulation, and calorie burn—tools that help you navigate plateaus and maintain momentum throughout your 21-day challenge.

HERBAL INFUSIONS & FUNCTIONAL TEA PAIRINGS

When you think of pink salt rituals, you might picture salt dissolved in water first thing in the morning. Yet pairing your elixir with a targeted herbal infusion or functional tea elevates the practice—adding plant compounds that support digestion, calm the nervous system, or gently boost metabolism. By weaving in different brews, you transform a simple drink into a personalized tonic ritual, tailored to your needs on any given day.

Choosing Herbs for Your Goals

Every herb carries its own profile of bioactive compounds. To select the right infusion, match the herb's traditional uses to your current priorities: digestion, stress relief, or metabolic support.

- Chamomile soothes the stomach and calms the mind, making it ideal for mornings after restless nights.

- Peppermint energizes digestion and freshens breath—perfect for days when you plan a larger lunch or anticipate heavy meals.
- \<Rhodiola rosea supports mild stress adaptation, helping you stay focused during back-to-back work calls.\</Rhodiola rosea>
- Green tea delivers a gentle caffeine lift plus catechins, which studies link to modest increases in fat oxidation.
- Rooibos offers antioxidants without caffeine, lending a slightly sweet, nutty flavor that complements salt's minerality.

To start, identify your top two concerns. If afternoon slumps and stress are your main obstacles, combine peppermint for digestion and Rhodiola for focus. If digestion and energy both feel low, a green tea pairing provides dual benefits.

Brewing Techniques That Preserve Potency

Not all infusions are created equal. Water temperature, steep time, and vessel material influence the extraction of active compounds. For most herbal tisanes, use water just below boiling (around 200°F) and steep for five to seven minutes. For green tea, lower the heat to about 175°F and limit steeping to two to three minutes to avoid bitterness.

- Herb-to-water ratio: one teaspoon of dried herb (or one teabag) per eight ounces of water.
- Steep in glass or ceramic—avoid reactive metals that can dull flavor and neutralize delicate compounds.
- Cover the cup to trap volatile oils during steeping, then strain or remove the teabag before adding pink salt elixir.

For example, if you choose peppermint, pour water over the leaves, cover, and steep for six minutes. Meanwhile, measure your pink salt and have it ready. After straining the infusion into your mug, stir in the salt, then sip slowly—allowing the minty steam to mingle with salt's subtle tang.

Sample Pairings and Their Effects

Pairing your elixir with functional brews becomes a creative ritual. Rotate these combinations through your week to keep your palate engaged and your body responsive.

- Day 1: Chamomile infusion + pink salt. Use post-elixir to settle the stomach and ease any tension after busy mornings.
- Day 2: Green tea + pink salt. Drink before activity to harness caffeine and catechins for low-level fat oxidation during your walk.
- Day 3: Peppermint tea + pink salt. Sip mid-morning to support digestion and refresh the palate after breakfast.
- Day 4: Rooibos + pink salt. Opt for this caffeine-free brew on heavy-meal days to introduce antioxidants without overstimulation.

- Day 5: Rhodiola tonic (steep Rhodiola root) + elixir. Combine with salt after a stressful morning to maintain focus through deadlines.
- Day 6: Hibiscus tea + pink salt. Hibiscus supports healthy blood pressure—ideal on high-sodium meal days to balance your system.
- Day 7: Your favorite infusion + pink salt. Reflect on the week and choose the brew you most enjoyed.

Each pairing addresses a different need while reinforcing the ritual's core: hydration, mineral balance, and habit consistency. By Day 7, you'll have a sense of which brews resonate most with your body and mood cycles.

Adjusting Based on Feedback

As with any experiment, pay close attention to subtle shifts. Keep brief journal notes:

- How does each pairing affect digestion? Note any bloating or comfort changes.
- Track mid-afternoon energy or focus after energizing teas versus calming infusions.
- Observe sleep quality if you use mild stimulants like green tea or Rhodiola in the morning.

If peppermint leaves you jittery, switch to chamomile for mid-morning. If rooibos feels too mild, try a half–green tea, half–rooibos blend. Over three weeks, you'll build a personalized roster of infusions that support your unique pattern of needs—digestive, cognitive, or stress-related.

Combining herbal infusions and functional teas with your pink salt ritual deepens each sip into a purposeful practice. By selecting herbs that target specific goals, mastering proper brewing, and rotating pairings based on personal feedback, you ensure the ritual remains engaging, effective, and aligned with your evolving challenges.

INTEGRATING LIGHT MOVEMENT & BREATHWORK

Introducing light movement and breathwork into your pink salt ritual transforms a simple morning sip into a full mind-body tune-up. By combining gentle physical activity with intentional breathing, you leverage two powerful systems: the musculoskeletal network that supports circulation and the autonomic nervous system that governs stress response. These additions amplify the benefits of hydration and electrolytes, helping you feel both grounded and energized.

Why Movement Matters First Thing

After hours of sleep, your body transitions from rest mode to wakefulness. Muscles can feel stiff, circulation slower, and joints less fluid. Incorporating light movement immediately after your pink salt elixir jump-starts the lymphatic system, enhances nutrient delivery, and primes muscles for the day ahead. You don't need a full workout—just enough to awaken your body.

- Joint lubrication: gentle dynamic stretches—pendulum swings for hips and shoulder circles—help synovial fluid distribute evenly.
- Circulation boost: movements like marching in place send fresh blood to extremities, increasing oxygen flow to cells.
- Activation of core muscles: simple toe lifts or seated pelvic tilts engage deep stabilizers, supporting posture throughout the day.

For example, stand beside your kitchen counter after stirring your elixir. Hold the edge lightly for balance and perform ten slow hip circles in each direction. Then lift onto your toes ten times, pressing down through heels on the return. These small actions mobilize joints and wake up the nervous system without causing fatigue.

Breathwork to Calm and Focus

Breath connects mind and body through the vagus nerve, which regulates heart rate, digestion, and stress responses. Intentional breath patterns can shift you from a reactive, fight-or-flight state into a more relaxed, focused mode—ideal for tackling work tasks or family routines.

Begin with three rounds of box breathing:

- Inhale through the nose for a count of four, feeling ribs expand.
- Hold gently for four counts, maintaining calm awareness.
- Exhale slowly for four counts, releasing tension.
- Pause for four counts before the next inhale.

This cycle resets cortisol levels and sharpens attention. Over weeks, you'll notice that brief morning breathwork reduces impulsive caffeine reaches and prevents that mid-morning energy crash. As you sip your pink salt water, breathe slowly, matching the rhythm of your stir to your inhale-exhale pattern—binding the habit together.

Sequencing Movement and Breath

The order of light movement and breathwork influences outcomes. Consider these sequences and choose the one that aligns with your goals:

- Movement first, then breathwork: mobilizes stiff joints, then calms the mind—ideal for mornings when you feel sluggish.
- Breathwork first, then movement: centers the mind before activating the body—helpful when anxiety or mind-racing greets you at dawn.
- Interleaved pattern: one minute of movement followed by one minute of breathwork, repeated three times—balances stimulation and relaxation.

If stress greets you before your feet even hit the floor, start with box breathing while seated, then transition into hip circles and toe raises. If your body feels stiff and tangled, perform the movement first, then settle into longer pranayama holds—like a six-second inhale and eight-second exhale—to soak in the physical activation.

Case Example: A Busy Morning Routine

Emily, our marketing manager, often feels overwhelmed by 7 a.m. panics—emails pinging, children calling for breakfast. She experimented with a brief practice: after stirring her pink salt drink, she stood beside her counter and did ten shoulder rolls backward and forward. Then, she closed her eyes for box breathing. Within five minutes, she reported feeling less reactive and more able to coach her kids through their morning without snapping at minor delays.

Practical Tips for Consistency

To weave movement and breath into your ritual seamlessly, follow these tips:

- Pair with a cue: link the start of breathing to the moment you finish stirring your elixir.
- Keep it short: aim for five total minutes—long enough for effect, short enough to fit any schedule.
- Use visual reminders: place a small yoga mat near your pink salt station or a sticky note on your mirror saying "Breathe & Move."
- Track your practice: in your journal or app, note what sequence you used and any immediate effects on mood or stiffness.

These strategies ensure practice survives even hectic days. If you miss the morning window due to an emergency, schedule a one-minute breath break at lunch or a brief stretch session before dinner—preserving the mind-body connection.

Expanding Over Three Weeks

As you progress through the 21-day challenge, gradually enhance your light movement and breathwork:

- Week 1: Master the basic sequence—three minutes of simple movement followed by two minutes of box breathing.
- Week 2: Experiment with varied breath techniques—try alternate nostril breathing (nadi shodhana) or a 4-7-8 pattern for deeper relaxation.
- Week 3: Add one new movement—such as gentle spinal twists or chair-supported squats—to increase mobility and metabolic engagement.

By Day 21, you'll carry a personalized blend of hydration, movement, and breath that opens your body, settles your mind, and amplifies every benefit of the pink salt ritual.

CHAPTER 4

Breakfast Recipes

Pink Salt Citrus Sunrise Elixir

Preparation Time: 5 minutes   **Cooking Time:** 0 minutes   **Servings:** 1

INGREDIENTS

- Water (8 fl oz, warm)
- Himalayan pink salt (¼ tsp)
- Lemon juice (1 tbsp, freshly squeezed)
- Orange juice (2 tbsp, freshly squeezed)
- Lemon zest (¼ tsp)
- Honey (1 tsp, optional)

PREPARATION

1. Pour 8 fl oz of warm water into a glass or mug.
2. Add ¼ tsp of Himalayan pink salt and stir until fully dissolved.
3. Squeeze 1 tbsp of fresh lemon juice and 2 tbsp of fresh orange juice into the glass.
4. Stir in ¼ tsp of lemon zest, ensuring it disperses evenly.
5. If desired, add 1 tsp of honey and mix until combined.

Benefits: This elixir delivers rapid hydration with electrolytes from pink salt and natural minerals that help balance fluids and support muscle function. The citrus provides a boost of vitamin C for immune health and antioxidants that fight free radicals. Morning consumption can improve digestion, enhance nutrient absorption, and gently stimulate metabolism. The combination of lemon zest and orange adds mood-lifting aroma, helping you feel refreshed, alert, and ready for the day.

Mineral-Infused Green Smoothie Bowl

Preparation Time: 10 minutes | **Cooking Time:** 0 minutes | **Servings:** 1

INGREDIENTS

- Frozen banana (1 medium, sliced)
- Baby spinach (1 cup, packed)
- Almond milk (½ cup, unsweetened)
- Greek yogurt (¼ cup, plain)
- Himalayan pink salt (⅛ tsp)
- Chia seeds (1 tbsp)
- Toppings: sliced kiwi (½ fruit), granola (2 tbsp), pumpkin seeds (1 tbsp)

PREPARATION

1. Combine frozen banana, baby spinach, almond milk, Greek yogurt, and ⅛ tsp pink salt in a blender.
2. Blend on high until thick and creamy, adding a splash of almond milk if needed for texture.
3. Pour the smoothie into a bowl and sprinkle 1 tbsp chia seeds evenly over the top.
4. Arrange sliced kiwi, 2 tbsp granola, and 1 tbsp pumpkin seeds in sections on the surface.

Benefits: This green smoothie bowl hydrates and replenishes electrolytes with pink salt while delivering fiber from banana and chia seeds for digestive support. Spinach provides iron and magnesium, key for energy production and muscle recovery. Greek yogurt adds protein to promote fullness and stabilize blood sugar. Toppings supply healthy fats and antioxidants, making this meal a nutrient-packed start that sustains energy through busy mornings.

Savory Pink Salt & Herb Avocado Toast

Preparation Time: 5 minutes | **Cooking Time:** 5 minutes | **Servings:** 1

INGREDIENTS

- Whole-grain bread (1 slice)
- Avocado (½ medium, ripe)
- Himalayan pink salt (¼ tsp)
- Fresh lemon juice (½ tsp)
- Fresh basil leaves (3 leaves, chopped)
- Fresh chives (1 tsp, minced)
- Cracked black pepper (to taste)
- Olive oil (½ tsp, optional)

PREPARATION

1. Toast 1 slice of whole-grain bread until golden brown.
2. In a small bowl, mash ½ avocado with ¼ tsp pink salt and ½ tsp lemon juice until creamy.
3. Spread the avocado mixture evenly over the toasted bread.
4. Sprinkle chopped basil, minced chives, and cracked black pepper over the top.
5. Drizzle ½ tsp olive oil if desired for extra richness.

Benefits: This avocado toast combines healthy monounsaturated fats for heart health with fiber to support steady digestion. Pink salt enhances mineral balance and adds depth of flavor, while lemon juice brightens the dish and aids nutrient absorption. Fresh herbs contribute antioxidants and natural phytochemicals that reduce inflammation. Together, these elements create a satisfying breakfast that nourishes the body and keeps you full until lunchtime.

Spiced Chia Pudding with Pink Salt Drizzle

Preparation Time: 5 minutes

Cooking Time: 0 minutes
(plus overnight chilling)

Servings: 2

INGREDIENTS

- Chia seeds (¼ cup)
- Almond milk (1 cup, unsweetened)
- Vanilla extract (½ tsp)
- Ground cinnamon (¼ tsp)
- Maple syrup (1 tbsp)
- Himalayan pink salt (⅛ tsp)
- Toppings: fresh berries (½ cup) and chopped nuts (2 tbsp)

PREPARATION

1. In a bowl, whisk together ¼ cup chia seeds, 1 cup almond milk, ½ tsp vanilla extract, ¼ tsp ground cinnamon, 1 tbsp maple syrup, and ⅛ tsp pink salt.
2. Cover and refrigerate for at least four hours or overnight, stirring once after an hour to prevent clumps.
3. After chilling, stir the pudding to achieve a uniform consistency.
4. Divide into two serving jars and top each with ¼ cup fresh berries and 1 tbsp chopped nuts.

Benefits: Chia pudding provides sustained energy through slow-digesting fiber and plant-based protein, supporting stable blood sugar. Pink salt in the mixture ensures balanced electrolytes for hydration and muscle function. Cinnamon adds compounds that may help regulate insulin response, while berries and nuts contribute antioxidants and healthy fats. This make-ahead breakfast saves time and delivers a nutrient-dense start to your day.

Protein-Packed Pink Salt Oat Pancakes

Preparation Time: 10 minutes

Cooking Time: 10 minutes

Servings: 2

INGREDIENTS

- Rolled oats (1 cup)
- Egg (1 large)
- Greek yogurt (¼ cup, plain)
- Milk (¼ cup, any variety)
- Baking powder (½ tsp)
- Himalayan pink salt (⅛ tsp)
- Vanilla extract (½ tsp)
- Cooking oil (1 tsp)

PREPARATION

1. Blend 1 cup rolled oats in a blender until fine, then transfer to a bowl.
2. Stir in ½ tsp baking powder and ⅛ tsp pink salt.
3. In a separate bowl, whisk 1 egg, ¼ cup Greek yogurt, ¼ cup milk, and ½ tsp vanilla extract.
4. Combine wet and dry ingredients until smooth.
5. Heat 1 tsp oil in a nonstick skillet over medium heat; pour ¼ cup batter for each pancake. Cook 2–3 minutes per side until golden.

Benefits: These pancakes blend whole-grain oats for fiber with Greek yogurt and egg for complete protein, promoting muscle repair and prolonged fullness. Pink salt adds essential minerals and balances fluid levels. Baking powder gives a light texture without excess sugar. This breakfast supports sustained energy and helps curb mid-morning cravings, ideal for active mornings or busy workdays.

Energizing Beet & Berry Power Parfait

Preparation Time: 10 minutes | **Cooking Time:** 0 minutes | **Servings:** 1

INGREDIENTS

- Cooked beets (¼ cup, diced)
- Mixed berries (½ cup, fresh or thawed)
- Greek yogurt (1 cup, plain)
- Himalayan pink salt (⅛ tsp)
- Honey (1 tbsp)
- Granola (2 tbsp)
- Fresh mint leaves (2, chopped)

PREPARATION

1. In a serving glass, layer ½ cup Greek yogurt at the bottom.
2. Sprinkle ⅛ tsp pink salt over the yogurt and drizzle with 1 tbsp honey.
3. Add a layer of ¼ cup diced cooked beets, followed by ½ cup mixed berries.
4. Top with 2 tbsp granola and garnish with chopped mint leaves.

Benefits: This parfait combines beets rich in nitrates for blood flow support with antioxidant-packed berries to protect cells from oxidative stress. Greek yogurt provides protein and probiotics for gut health, while pink salt replenishes electrolytes. Honey offers natural sweetness and quick energy without spikes. The result is a colorful, nutrient-dense breakfast that boosts circulation, supports digestion, and keeps you energized through morning tasks.

Pink Salt Yogurt Parfait with Nuts & Seeds

Preparation Time: 5 minutes | **Cooking Time:** 0 minutes | **Servings:** 1

INGREDIENTS

- Greek yogurt (1 cup, plain)
- Himalayan pink salt (⅛ tsp)
- Raw almonds (2 tbsp, chopped)
- Raw pumpkin seeds (1 tbsp)
- Chia seeds (1 tbsp)
- Honey (1 tsp)
- Fresh berries (¼ cup, mixed)

PREPARATION

1. Spoon ½ cup Greek yogurt into a tall glass or bowl.
2. Sprinkle ⅛ tsp pink salt over the yogurt and drizzle with 1 tsp honey.
3. Layer 2 tbsp chopped almonds and 1 tbsp pumpkin seeds on top.
4. Add the remaining ½ cup yogurt, then scatter 1 tbsp chia seeds.
5. Top with ¼ cup fresh berries and serve immediately.

Benefits: This parfait delivers a balance of protein and healthy fats to stabilize blood sugar and curb mid-morning hunger. Pink salt adds trace minerals that support hydration and nerve function. Nuts and seeds bring vitamin E, magnesium, and omega-3s for brain and heart health, while chia seeds provide fiber for digestive regularity. The fresh berries contribute antioxidants, making this a nutrient-dense breakfast that fuels both body and mind. (#ni#)

Zesty Pink Salt Veggie Frittata

Preparation Time: 10 minutes   **Cooking Time:** 15 minutes   **Servings:** 2

INGREDIENTS

- Eggs (4 large)
- Himalayan pink salt (¼ tsp)
- Black pepper (to taste)
- Olive oil (1 tbsp)
- Onion (¼ cup, diced)
- Bell pepper (¼ cup, diced)
- Zucchini (¼ cup, sliced)
- Cherry tomatoes (¼ cup, halved)
- Fresh parsley (1 tbsp, chopped)

PREPARATION

1. Preheat oven to 350°F and heat 1 tbsp olive oil in an ovenproof skillet over medium heat.
2. Sauté ¼ cup onion, ¼ cup bell pepper, and ¼ cup zucchini until soft, about 5 minutes.
3. In a bowl, whisk 4 eggs with ¼ tsp pink salt and black pepper.
4. Pour the egg mixture over the vegetables, scatter ¼ cup cherry tomatoes, and cook without stirring for 2 minutes.
5. Transfer skillet to oven and bake for 10–12 minutes until set. Garnish with 1 tbsp parsley.

Benefits: This frittata combines high-quality protein from eggs with fiber and phyto-nutrients from vegetables, creating a filling breakfast that supports muscle health and digestion. Pink salt enhances electrolyte balance, aiding muscle function and preventing cramps. Fresh parsley adds vitamins A and C, promoting immune function. Baked rather than fried, this dish packs savory flavor without excess oil, keeping calories in check while delivering sustained energy.

Quinoa Porridge with Pink Salt & Cinnamon

Preparation Time: 5 minutes   **Cooking Time:** 20 minutes   **Servings:** 2

INGREDIENTS

- Quinoa (½ cup, rinsed)
- Water (1 cup)
- Milk (1 cup, any variety)
- Himalayan pink salt (⅛ tsp)
- Ground cinnamon (½ tsp)
- Maple syrup (2 tsp)
- Sliced banana (1 medium)

PREPARATION

1. Combine ½ cup rinsed quinoa and 1 cup water in a saucepan; bring to a boil.
2. Reduce heat, cover, and simmer 15 minutes until water is absorbed.
3. Stir in 1 cup milk, ⅛ tsp pink salt, and ½ tsp cinnamon; simmer 5 more minutes.
4. Divide porridge between bowls, drizzle 2 tsp maple syrup, and top with sliced banana.

Benefits: Quinoa provides complete plant protein and fiber for lasting fullness and stable blood sugar. Pink salt contributes essential minerals for hydration and metabolism. Cinnamon offers compounds that may support insulin sensitivity and add warm flavor without extra sugar. Combined with natural sweetness from maple syrup and banana, this porridge nourishes muscles, supports digestion, and supplies gentle energy for a productive morning.

Tropical Coconut-Pink Salt Smoothie

Preparation Time: 5 minutes   **Cooking Time:** 0 minutes   **Servings:** 1

INGREDIENTS

- Frozen pineapple chunks (½ cup)
- Frozen mango chunks (½ cup)
- Coconut water (1 cup)
- Himalayan pink salt (⅛ tsp)
- Greek yogurt (2 tbsp, plain)
- Fresh lime juice (1 tsp)
- Shredded coconut (1 tsp, for garnish)

PREPARATION

1. Place ½ cup pineapple, ½ cup mango, 1 cup coconut water, and ⅛ tsp pink salt in a blender.
2. Add 2 tbsp Greek yogurt and 1 tsp lime juice.
3. Blend on high until smooth and creamy.
4. Pour into a glass and sprinkle 1 tsp shredded coconut on top.

Benefits: This smoothie hydrates quickly with coconut water's electrolytes and boosts mineral intake via pink salt. Tropical fruits deliver vitamins A and C, supporting immune health and skin. Greek yogurt adds protein for satiety, while lime juice aids digestion and refreshes the palate. The combination energizes with natural sugars and sustains you through morning tasks without a sugar crash.

Pink Salt Scrambled Egg Muffins

Preparation Time: 10 minutes   **Cooking Time:** 20 minutes   **Servings:** 6 muffins

INGREDIENTS

- Eggs (6 large)
- Himalayan pink salt (¼ tsp)
- Black pepper (to taste)
- Cheddar cheese (¼ cup, shredded)
- Baby spinach (½ cup, chopped)
- Bell pepper (¼ cup, diced)
- Olive oil (1 tsp, for greasing)

PREPARATION

1. Preheat oven to 350°F and grease a 6-cup muffin tin with 1 tsp olive oil.
2. In a bowl, whisk 6 eggs with ¼ tsp pink salt and black pepper.
3. Stir in ¼ cup cheese, ½ cup spinach, and ¼ cup bell pepper.
4. Divide mixture evenly among muffin cups.
5. Bake 18–20 minutes until set and lightly golden.

Benefits: These muffins deliver portable protein and vegetables in one grab-and-go package, supporting muscle repair and nutrient intake. Pink salt adds electrolytes to help maintain fluid balance and prevent cramps. Spinach and bell pepper provide vitamins and antioxidants to reduce inflammation and support immunity. Perfect for busy mornings, they ensure you start the day with a well-rounded, satisfying meal.

Almond-Flour Pink Salt Waffles

Preparation Time: 10 minutes　　**Cooking Time:** 10 minutes　　**Servings:** 2 waffles

INGREDIENTS

- Almond flour (½ cup)
- Egg (1 large)
- Unsweetened almond milk (2 tbsp)
- Baking powder (¼ tsp)
- Himalayan pink salt (⅛ tsp)
- Vanilla extract (¼ tsp)
- Coconut oil (for greasing)

PREPARATION

1. Preheat waffle iron and lightly grease with coconut oil.
2. In a bowl, whisk ½ cup almond flour, ¼ tsp baking powder, and ⅛ tsp pink salt.
3. In another bowl, beat 1 egg with 2 tbsp almond milk and ¼ tsp vanilla extract.
4. Combine wet and dry ingredients until a smooth batter forms.
5. Pour batter into the heated waffle iron and cook according to manufacturer's instructions (about 4–5 minutes) until golden.

Benefits: These grain-free waffles provide healthy fats and protein from almond flour and egg, helping to stabilize blood sugar and support muscle maintenance. Pink salt supplies trace minerals that aid hydration and nerve function. Lightly sweet and crisp, they satisfy a waffle craving without the carb overload, making them suitable for low-glycemic meal plans and busy mornings.

Pink Salt Overnight Oats with Fruit

Preparation Time: 5 minutes　　**Cooking Time:** 0 minutes (overnight chill)　　**Servings:** 1

INGREDIENTS

- Rolled oats (½ cup)
- Milk (¾ cup, any variety)
- Chia seeds (1 tbsp)
- Himalayan pink salt (⅛ tsp)
- Maple syrup (1 tsp)
- Mixed fruit (½ cup, diced; e.g., apple, berries)

PREPARATION

1. In a jar or bowl, combine ½ cup rolled oats, ¾ cup milk, 1 tbsp chia seeds, and ⅛ tsp pink salt.
2. Stir in 1 tsp maple syrup until well mixed.
3. Cover and refrigerate overnight (at least eight hours).
4. In the morning, give the oats a stir, top with ½ cup diced mixed fruit, and enjoy chilled.

Benefits: Overnight oats deliver slow-release carbohydrates and fiber to keep you full and energized through the morning. Pink salt ensures balanced electrolytes for hydration and supports digestive comfort. Chia seeds add additional fiber and omega-3s, promoting healthy digestion and heart health. Topped with fresh fruit, this breakfast provides vitamins, antioxidants, and natural sweetness in a ready-to-eat format for busy routines.

Savory Sweet Potato & Pink Salt Hash

Preparation Time: 10 minutes   **Cooking Time:** 15 minutes   **Servings:** 2

INGREDIENTS

- Sweet potato (1 medium, peeled and diced)
- Olive oil (1 tbsp)
- Onion (¼ cup, diced)
- Bell pepper (¼ cup, diced)
- Garlic (1 clove, minced)
- Himalayan pink salt (¼ tsp)
- Black pepper (to taste)
- Fresh cilantro (1 tbsp, chopped)

PREPARATION

1. Heat 1 tbsp olive oil in a large skillet over medium heat.
2. Add diced sweet potato and cook 5 minutes, stirring occasionally.
3. Stir in ¼ cup onion, ¼ cup bell pepper, and 1 clove minced garlic; cook another 5–7 minutes until vegetables are tender.
4. Season with ¼ tsp pink salt and black pepper, mixing thoroughly.
5. Remove from heat, sprinkle 1 tbsp chopped cilantro, and serve hot.

Benefits: This hash combines complex carbohydrates from sweet potato with protein-supporting herbs and vegetables to provide sustained energy. Pink salt replenishes essential minerals lost during overnight fasting and supports fluid balance. Bell pepper and onion add vitamins A and C, promoting immune function, while cilantro offers antioxidants. Enjoying this savory dish early helps regulate blood sugar and curbs mid-morning cravings.

Pink Salt Kefir Breakfast Bowl

Preparation Time: 5 minutes   **Cooking Time:** 0 minutes   **Servings:** 1

INGREDIENTS

- Plain kefir (1 cup)
- Himalayan pink salt (⅛ tsp)
- Rolled oats (2 tbsp)
- Fresh strawberries (¼ cup, sliced)
- Banana (½ medium, sliced)
- Almond butter (1 tsp)
- Hemp seeds (1 tsp)

PREPARATION

1. Pour 1 cup plain kefir into a bowl and stir in ⅛ tsp pink salt.
2. Sprinkle 2 tbsp rolled oats over the kefir and let sit one minute to soften.
3. Arrange ¼ cup sliced strawberries and ½ banana slices on top.
4. Drizzle 1 tsp almond butter and scatter 1 tsp hemp seeds as garnish.

Benefits: Kefir provides probiotics to support gut microbiota and digestion, complemented by electrolytes from pink salt for hydration. Oats supply fiber for fullness, while fruit adds natural sugars and antioxidants that support immune health. Almond butter brings healthy fats and protein, and hemp seeds contribute plant-based omega-3s. This breakfast bowl aids digestion, stabilizes blood sugar, and delivers a creamy, tangy, nourishing start to your day.

CHAPTER 5

Lunch Recipes

Pink Salt Citrus Quinoa Salad

Preparation Time: 15 minutes   **Cooking Time:** 15 minutes   **Servings:** 2

INGREDIENTS

- Quinoa (½ cup, rinsed)
- Water (1 cup)
- Himalayan pink salt (¼ tsp)
- Olive oil (1 tbsp, extra-virgin)
- Orange (1 medium, segmented and juice reserved)
- Grapefruit (½ medium, segmented and juice reserved)
- Cucumber (½ cup, diced)
- Red bell pepper (½ cup, diced)
- Fresh mint (2 tbsp, chopped)
- Fresh parsley (2 tbsp, chopped)
- Red onion (2 tbsp, finely minced)
- Lemon juice (1 tbsp, freshly squeezed)
- Black pepper (to taste)

PREPARATION

1. In a small saucepan, combine ½ cup rinsed quinoa, 1 cup water, and ¼ tsp Himalayan pink salt; bring to a boil.
2. Reduce heat to low, cover, and simmer for 12–15 minutes until quinoa absorbs the water and appears translucent.
3. While quinoa cooks, place orange and grapefruit segments in a bowl and squeeze leftover membranes to collect any remaining juice.
4. Transfer cooked quinoa to a large mixing bowl and let cool slightly, about 5 minutes.
5. Whisk together 1 tbsp olive oil, 1 tbsp lemon juice, reserved citrus juices, and a pinch of black pepper.
6. Add diced cucumber, red bell pepper, minced red onion, chopped mint, and parsley to the quinoa.
7. Pour the citrus–olive oil dressing over the quinoa mixture and gently toss to combine all ingredients.
8. Fold in the citrus segments last to preserve their shape, then taste and adjust seasoning with additional pink salt or pepper if needed.

Benefits: This salad delivers plant-based protein and fiber from quinoa, supporting digestive health and steady energy release. Himalayan pink salt supplies trace minerals and helps maintain fluid balance. Citrus fruits contribute vitamin C and antioxidants that boost immune function and collagen production, while olive oil provides heart-healthy monounsaturated fats. Fresh herbs and vegetables add phytonutrients and further fiber, making this dish a vibrant, hydrating lunch that nourishes the body and satisfies the palate.

Grilled Chicken & Pink Salt Veggie Wrap

Preparation Time: 15 minutes   **Cooking Time:** 12 minutes   **Servings:** 2

INGREDIENTS

- Boneless, skinless chicken breast (8 oz)
- Himalayan pink salt (¼ tsp)
- Black pepper (to taste)
- Olive oil (1 tbsp)
- Whole-wheat tortilla wraps (2 large)
- Mixed salad greens (1 cup)
- Cucumber (½ cup, thinly sliced)
- Bell pepper (½ cup, thinly sliced)
- Carrot (¼ cup, shredded)
- Hummus (2 tbsp)
- Lemon juice (1 tsp, optional)

PREPARATION

1. Season 8 oz chicken breast with ¼ tsp pink salt and black pepper; drizzle with 1 tbsp olive oil and rub evenly.
2. Heat a grill pan over medium-high heat; grill chicken 5–6 minutes per side until cooked through and juices run clear.
3. Transfer chicken to a cutting board and let rest 5 minutes, then slice into thin strips.
4. Warm 2 tortilla wraps in the pan for 30 seconds each side.
5. Spread 1 tbsp hummus in the center of each wrap and drizzle 1 tsp lemon juice if using.
6. Layer ½ cup mixed greens, ¼ cup cucumber, ¼ cup bell pepper, 2 tbsp shredded carrot, and half the chicken strips.
7. Fold in the sides of the wrap and roll tightly; cut in half on a diagonal and serve.

Benefits: This wrap combines lean protein from grilled chicken with the hydrating and mineral benefits of pink salt, supporting muscle repair and electrolyte balance. Whole-wheat tortillas and vegetables add fiber for digestion and sustained energy. Hummus contributes plant protein and healthy fats that stabilize blood sugar, while fresh veggies supply vitamins and antioxidants to enhance immunity and skin health. Perfect for a portable lunch that nourishes and satisfies.

Mediterranean Chickpea & Pink Salt Salad

Preparation Time: 10 minutes　　**Cooking Time:** 0 minutes　　**Servings:** 2

INGREDIENTS

- Chickpeas (1½ cups, cooked or canned, drained)
- Cucumber (1 cup, diced)
- Cherry tomatoes (1 cup, halved)
- Red onion (¼ cup, finely diced)
- Kalamata olives (¼ cup, pitted and sliced)
- Feta cheese (¼ cup, crumbled)
- Himalayan pink salt (½ tsp)
- Olive oil (2 tbsp)
- Red wine vinegar (1 tbsp)
- Dried oregano (½ tsp)
- Fresh parsley (2 tbsp, chopped)

PREPARATION

1. In a large mixing bowl, combine 1½ cups chickpeas, 1 cup cucumber, 1 cup cherry tomatoes, ¼ cup red onion, and ¼ cup olives.
2. Drizzle with 2 tbsp olive oil and 1 tbsp red wine vinegar.
3. Sprinkle ½ tsp pink salt and ½ tsp dried oregano over the salad.
4. Toss gently to coat all ingredients in the dressing.
5. Fold in ¼ cup crumbled feta and 2 tbsp chopped parsley just before serving.

Benefits: This salad blends fiber-rich chickpeas with hydrating vegetables, promoting digestive regularity and fluid balance. Pink salt supports electrolyte replenishment, while olive oil and olives provide heart-healthy monounsaturated fats. Feta cheese offers calcium and a savory punch, and herbs add antioxidants for inflammation control. The result is a vibrant, protein-rich lunch that sustains energy and supports overall wellness.

Pink Salt–Seasoned Salmon with Greens

Preparation Time: 10 minutes　　**Cooking Time:** 15 minutes　　**Servings:** 2

INGREDIENTS

- Salmon fillets (2 × 4 oz)
- Himalayan pink salt (½ tsp)
- Black pepper (to taste)
- Olive oil (1 tbsp)
- Lemon slices (4, for garnish)
- Mixed baby greens (4 cups)
- Cherry tomatoes (½ cup, halved)
- Cucumber (½ cup, sliced)
- Balsamic vinaigrette (2 tbsp)

PREPARATION

1. Preheat oven to 400°F and line a baking sheet with foil.
2. Place 2 salmon fillets on the sheet, drizzle with 1 tbsp olive oil, and season with ½ tsp pink salt and pepper.
3. Bake salmon 12–15 minutes until it flakes easily with a fork.
4. Meanwhile, toss 4 cups greens, ½ cup cherry tomatoes, and ½ cup cucumber with 2 tbsp vinaigrette in a large bowl.
5. Transfer greens to serving plates, top each with a salmon fillet, and garnish with 2 lemon slices.

Benefits: Salmon provides omega-3 fatty acids and high-quality protein, supporting brain and cardiovascular health. Pink salt ensures balanced electrolytes and enhances flavor without excess sodium. Mixed greens contribute vitamins A and K for bone and eye health, while tomatoes and cucumbers add hydration and antioxidants. This balanced plate fuels recovery, sharpens focus, and sustains energy through afternoon activities.

Zoodle Salad with Pink Salt Vinaigrette

Preparation Time: 15 minutes   **Cooking Time:** 0 minutes   **Servings:** 2

INGREDIENTS

- Zucchini (2 medium, spiralized)
- Cherry tomatoes (1 cup, quartered)
- Avocado (1 medium, diced)
- Red onion (2 tbsp, thinly sliced)
- Himalayan pink salt (½ tsp)
- Olive oil (2 tbsp)
- Lemon juice (1 tbsp, freshly squeezed)
- Fresh basil (2 tbsp, chopped)
- Parmesan cheese (2 tbsp, shaved, optional)

PREPARATION

1. Place 2 spiralized zucchinis in a large bowl and sprinkle with ½ tsp pink salt; toss and let sit 5 minutes to draw out water.
2. Drain excess liquid, then add 1 cup cherry tomatoes, 1 diced avocado, and 2 tbsp sliced red onion.
3. Whisk together 2 tbsp olive oil and 1 tbsp lemon juice.
4. Pour the vinaigrette over the salad and gently toss to coat.
5. Fold in 2 tbsp chopped basil and top with 2 tbsp shaved Parmesan if desired.

Benefits: Zoodles offer a low-carb alternative to pasta, providing hydration and fiber for digestion. Pink salt enhances mineral intake and elevates flavors. Olive oil and avocado deliver healthy fats that improve nutrient absorption and support satiety. Tomatoes and basil add antioxidants and anti-inflammatory compounds. This fresh, crisp salad keeps you feeling light and energized, perfect for a midday reset.

Turkey-Avocado Pink Salt Lettuce Cups

Preparation Time: 10 minutes   **Cooking Time:** 8 minutes   **Servings:** 2

INGREDIENTS

- Lean ground turkey (8 oz)
- Himalayan pink salt (¼ tsp)
- Black pepper (to taste)
- Garlic powder (½ tsp)
- Onion powder (½ tsp)
- Olive oil (1 tsp)
- Romaine lettuce leaves (8 large, rinsed)
- Avocado (1 medium, sliced)
- Cherry tomatoes (½ cup, quartered)
- Fresh cilantro (2 tbsp, chopped)
- Lime wedges (2, for serving)

PREPARATION

1. Heat 1 tsp olive oil in a skillet over medium heat.
2. Add 8 oz ground turkey, ¼ tsp pink salt, black pepper, ½ tsp garlic powder, and ½ tsp onion powder; cook 6–8 minutes, breaking up meat, until browned.
3. Remove skillet from heat and let turkey mixture rest one minute.
4. Arrange 8 lettuce leaves on a platter.
5. Spoon turkey filling evenly into each leaf, then top with sliced avocado and quartered cherry tomatoes.
6. Sprinkle 2 tbsp chopped cilantro over cups and serve with lime wedges.

Benefits: These lettuce cups deliver lean protein from turkey to support muscle repair and satiety, while pink salt replenishes essential electrolytes. Avocado provides heart-healthy monounsaturated fats, and tomatoes contribute vitamin C and antioxidants. Lettuce leaves offer hydration and fiber without added carbs. Together, these ingredients create a light yet satisfying lunch that stabilizes blood sugar and nourishes your body.

Pink Salt–Drizzled Sweet Potato Bowls

Preparation Time: 10 minutes   **Cooking Time:** 30 minutes   **Servings:** 2

INGREDIENTS

- Sweet potatoes (2 medium, scrubbed)
- Himalayan pink salt (½ tsp)
- Black pepper (to taste)
- Olive oil (1 tbsp)
- Kale (2 cups, chopped)
- Chickpeas (1 cup, cooked or canned, drained)
- Tahini (1 tbsp)
- Lemon juice (1 tsp)

PREPARATION

1. Preheat oven to 400°F. Pierce 2 sweet potatoes with a fork and bake 25–30 minutes until tender.
2. Meanwhile, toss 1 cup chickpeas with ¼ tsp pink salt and roast on a separate sheet for 15 minutes until crisp.
3. In a small bowl, whisk 1 tbsp tahini, 1 tsp lemon juice, and a pinch of black pepper; set aside.
4. Sauté 2 cups chopped kale in 1 tsp olive oil until wilted, about 3 minutes. Season with a pinch of pink salt.
5. Split baked potatoes, fluff insides with a fork, and drizzle 1 tbsp olive oil and ¼ tsp pink salt over each.
6. Top each potato with kale, roasted chickpeas, and drizzle with tahini sauce.

Benefits: This bowl combines complex carbs from sweet potato with protein and fiber from chickpeas, providing sustained energy. Pink salt enhances mineral balance, while kale adds vitamins A and K for bone and eye health. Tahini supplies calcium and healthy fats for nutrient absorption. The result is a hearty, nutrient-dense meal that supports digestion, hydration, and metabolic function.

Lentil & Pink Salt Soup

Preparation Time: 10 minutes **Cooking Time:** 30 minutes **Servings:** 4

INGREDIENTS

- Brown lentils (1 cup, rinsed)
- Water or vegetable broth (4 cups)
- Himalayan pink salt (½ tsp, plus extra to taste)
- Olive oil (1 tbsp)
- Carrot (1 medium, diced)
- Celery (1 stalk, diced)
- Onion (1 small, diced)
- Garlic (2 cloves, minced)
- Ground cumin (½ tsp)
- Smoked paprika (½ tsp)
- Fresh spinach (2 cups)
- Fresh parsley (2 tbsp, chopped)

PREPARATION

1. Heat 1 tbsp olive oil in a large pot over medium heat; sauté 1 small diced onion, 1 diced carrot, and 1 diced celery stalk for 5 minutes.
2. Add 2 minced garlic cloves, ½ tsp cumin, and ½ tsp smoked paprika; cook 1 minute until fragrant.
3. Stir in 1 cup lentils, 4 cups broth, and ½ tsp pink salt; bring to a boil.
4. Reduce heat, cover, and simmer 25 minutes until lentils are tender.
5. Stir in 2 cups spinach and cook 2 more minutes until wilted.
6. Taste and adjust seasoning with additional pink salt and pepper; garnish with 2 tbsp chopped parsley.

Benefits: Lentils offer plant protein and iron to support energy levels and muscle function, while dietary fiber promotes digestive health. Pink salt replaces essential minerals lost through fluid shifts. Aromatic spices add anti-inflammatory benefits and depth of flavor. Spinach introduces vitamins and antioxidants, making this soup a warming, nutrient-packed lunch that sustains fullness and supports your 21-day challenge.

Asian-Style Pink Salt Tofu Salad

Preparation Time: 15 minutes   **Cooking Time:** 10 minutes   **Servings:** 2

INGREDIENTS

- Firm tofu (8 oz, drained and cubed)
- Himalayan pink salt (¼ tsp)
- Black pepper (to taste)
- Sesame oil (1 tbsp)
- Rice vinegar (1 tbsp)
- Soy sauce (1 tsp, low-sodium)
- Cucumber (1 cup, julienned)
- Carrot (½ cup, julienned)
- Red cabbage (1 cup, shredded)
- Green onions (2, sliced)
- Sesame seeds (1 tsp)

PREPARATION

1. Heat 1 tbsp sesame oil in a nonstick pan; add 8 oz tofu cubes seasoned with ¼ tsp pink salt and pepper.
2. Cook tofu 4–5 minutes per side until golden brown.
3. Whisk 1 tbsp rice vinegar and 1 tsp soy sauce in a small bowl; set dressing aside.
4. In a large bowl, combine 1 cup cucumber, ½ cup carrot, and 1 cup cabbage.
5. Add cooked tofu and drizzle with dressing; toss gently to coat.
6. Garnish with sliced green onions and 1 tsp sesame seeds before serving.

Benefits: Tofu supplies complete plant protein and calcium for bone health, while pink salt provides trace minerals essential for nerve and muscle function. Sesame oil and seeds add healthy fats and antioxidants. Fresh vegetables contribute fiber, vitamins, and hydration. The tangy, umami dressing aids digestion, making this salad a balanced, flavorful lunch that supports your energy and wellness goals.

Pink Salt Quinoa-Stuffed Peppers

Preparation Time: 15 minutes   **Cooking Time:** 35 minutes   **Servings:** 4 peppers

INGREDIENTS

- Bell peppers (4 large, tops cut off, seeds removed)
- Quinoa (1 cup, rinsed and cooked)
- Himalayan pink salt (½ tsp)
- Black pepper (to taste)
- Olive oil (1 tbsp)
- Onion (½ cup, diced)
- Garlic (2 cloves, minced)
- Tomato (1 cup, diced)
- Black beans (1 cup, cooked or canned, drained)
- Cumin (½ tsp)
- Shredded cheddar cheese (½ cup)
- Fresh cilantro (2 tbsp, chopped)

PREPARATION

1. Preheat oven to 375°F and brush 4 bell peppers with 1 tsp olive oil inside and out.
2. In a skillet, heat remaining 2 tsp olive oil; sauté ½ cup onion and 2 minced garlic cloves for 3 minutes.
3. Stir in 1 cup diced tomato, 1 cup black beans, 1 cup cooked quinoa, ½ tsp cumin, ½ tsp pink salt, and pepper; cook 2 minutes.
4. Spoon quinoa mixture into each pepper, packing tightly.
5. Place stuffed peppers in a baking dish, cover with foil, and bake 25 minutes.
6. Remove foil, top each with 2 tbsp cheese, and bake 5 more minutes until cheese melts. Garnish with cilantro.

Benefits: These stuffed peppers blend complete protein from quinoa and beans with fiber and vitamins from peppers and tomatoes. Pink salt enhances mineral balance and flavor. Cheese adds calcium and protein, supporting bone and muscle health. Cilantro contributes antioxidants. This hearty, colorful dish delivers sustained energy, supports digestion, and satisfies mid-day hunger while fitting your 21-day plan.

Kale & Pink Salt Roasted Pepper Salad

Preparation Time: 10 minutes **Cooking Time:** 20 minutes **Servings:** 2

INGREDIENTS

- Kale (4 cups, stems removed and chopped)
- Red bell pepper (1 large, sliced)
- Yellow bell pepper (1 large, sliced)
- Olive oil (2 tbsp)
- Himalayan pink salt (½ tsp)
- Black pepper (to taste)
- Lemon juice (1 tbsp, freshly squeezed)
- Parmesan cheese (2 tbsp, grated)

PREPARATION

1. Preheat oven to 425°F and line a baking sheet with parchment.
2. Toss sliced red and yellow peppers with 1 tbsp olive oil, ¼ tsp pink salt, and pepper.
3. Roast peppers 15–20 minutes until tender and slightly charred, then let cool.
4. In a large bowl, massage 4 cups kale with remaining 1 tbsp olive oil, ¼ tsp pink salt, and 1 tbsp lemon juice until leaves soften.
5. Add roasted peppers to the kale and gently toss.
6. Sprinkle 2 tbsp grated Parmesan over the salad before serving.

Benefits: Kale provides a powerhouse of vitamins A, C, and K along with fiber that supports digestion and satiety. Roasted peppers supply antioxidants like beta-carotene, and olive oil helps absorb fat-soluble nutrients. Himalayan pink salt restores trace minerals for hydration and nerve function. The bright lemon juice enhances nutrient uptake, and Parmesan adds protein and calcium for bone health. This vibrant salad hydrates, nourishes, and keeps energy levels steady.

Pink Salt Tuna Salad with Apples

Preparation Time: 10 minutes **Cooking Time:** 0 minutes **Servings:** 2

INGREDIENTS

- Canned tuna (5 oz, drained)
- Himalayan pink salt (¼ tsp)
- Black pepper (to taste)
- Greek yogurt (2 tbsp, plain)
- Dijon mustard (1 tsp)
- Apple (½ medium, diced)
- Celery (¼ cup, diced)
- Red onion (2 tbsp, minced)
- Fresh dill (1 tbsp, chopped)
- Lemon juice (1 tsp)

PREPARATION

1. In a bowl, combine 5 oz drained tuna, 2 tbsp Greek yogurt, 1 tsp Dijon mustard, ¼ tsp pink salt, and pepper.
2. Stir in diced apple, celery, red onion, and 1 tsp lemon juice until evenly distributed.
3. Fold in chopped dill gently, keeping apple pieces intact.
4. Taste and adjust seasoning with additional pink salt or lemon juice if needed.
5. Serve on a bed of greens or in lettuce wraps.

Benefits: Tuna delivers lean protein and omega-3 fatty acids, supporting muscle repair and brain health. Apple adds fiber and natural sweetness, aiding digestion and blood sugar control. Himalayan pink salt ensures trace minerals for nerve and fluid balance. Greek yogurt provides probiotics for gut health, and dill brings antioxidants and flavor without added calories. This refreshing salad keeps you satisfied and supports metabolic balance.

Pink Salt Shrimp & Avocado Plate

Preparation Time: 10 minutes   **Cooking Time:** 8 minutes   **Servings:** 2

INGREDIENTS

- Shrimp (10 large, peeled and deveined)
- Himalayan pink salt (¼ tsp)
- Black pepper (to taste)
- Olive oil (1 tbsp)
- Avocado (1 medium, sliced)
- Cherry tomatoes (½ cup, halved)
- Cucumber (½ cup, sliced)
- Lime juice (1 tbsp, freshly squeezed)
- Fresh cilantro (1 tbsp, chopped)

PREPARATION

1. Season shrimp with ¼ tsp pink salt and pepper.
2. Heat 1 tbsp olive oil in a skillet over medium-high heat; cook shrimp 2–3 minutes per side until pink and opaque.
3. Arrange sliced avocado, tomatoes, and cucumber on a plate.
4. Place cooked shrimp atop the vegetables.
5. Drizzle 1 tbsp lime juice over the plate and sprinkle 1 tbsp chopped cilantro.
6. Serve immediately, enjoying warm shrimp with cool produce.

Benefits: Shrimp offers lean protein and selenium for immune health, while avocado delivers heart-healthy monounsaturated fats and potassium. Himalayan pink salt restores trace minerals essential for nerve and muscle function. Tomatoes and cucumber hydrate and provide antioxidants. Lime juice enhances flavor and vitamin C, aiding iron absorption. The combination creates a balanced, refreshing meal that supports satiety, hydration, and metabolic health.

Pink Salt–Roasted Cauliflower Bowls

Preparation Time: 10 minutes   **Cooking Time:** 25 minutes   **Servings:** 2

INGREDIENTS

- Cauliflower florets (4 cups)
- Olive oil (2 tbsp)
- Himalayan pink salt (½ tsp)
- Ground cumin (½ tsp)
- Paprika (½ tsp)
- Chickpeas (1 cup, cooked or canned, drained)
- Quinoa (1 cup, cooked)
- Baby spinach (1 cup)
- Tahini dressing (2 tbsp)

PREPARATION

1. Preheat oven to 425°F and line a baking sheet with parchment paper.
2. In a bowl, toss 4 cups cauliflower with 2 tbsp olive oil, ½ tsp pink salt, ½ tsp cumin, and ½ tsp paprika.
3. Spread seasoned cauliflower on the sheet and roast 20–25 minutes until tender and golden, stirring once at 10 minutes.
4. Warm 1 cup cooked chickpeas in a small pan with a pinch of pink salt if desired.
5. Divide 1 cup cooked quinoa and 1 cup baby spinach between two bowls.
6. Top each bowl with roasted cauliflower and chickpeas, then drizzle 1 tbsp tahini dressing over each.

Benefits: Roasted cauliflower provides fiber and vitamin C, while pink salt restores essential minerals lost overnight. Chickpeas and quinoa deliver complete plant protein and complex carbohydrates for lasting energy. Tahini adds calcium and healthy fats that support joint health and nutrient absorption. This balanced bowl keeps you full longer, aids digestion, and helps stabilize blood sugar, making it ideal for a nourishing midday meal.

Warm Farro & Pink Salt Veggie Medley

Preparation Time: 10 minutes   **Cooking Time:** 30 minutes   **Servings:** 2

INGREDIENTS

- Farro (½ cup, rinsed)
- Water or vegetable broth (1½ cups)
- Himalayan pink salt (½ tsp)
- Olive oil (1 tbsp)
- Zucchini (½ cup, diced)
- Carrot (½ cup, sliced)
- Broccoli florets (½ cup)
- Garlic (1 clove, minced)
- Lemon zest (½ tsp)
- Fresh parsley (1 tbsp, chopped)

PREPARATION

1. In a saucepan, bring 1½ cups water or broth and ½ tsp pink salt to a boil.
2. Add ½ cup farro, reduce heat, and simmer 25–30 minutes until tender; drain any excess liquid.
3. While farro cooks, heat 1 tbsp olive oil in a skillet over medium heat; sauté garlic 1 minute.
4. Add diced zucchini, carrot, and broccoli; cook 5–7 minutes until vegetables are crisp-tender.
5. Stir in cooked farro, ½ tsp lemon zest, and 1 tbsp parsley; toss to combine and warm through.
6. Adjust seasoning with additional pink salt and serve immediately.

Benefits: Farro is an ancient grain rich in fiber, protein, and minerals like magnesium for energy metabolism. The colorful vegetables supply vitamins, antioxidants, and phytonutrients that support immune and digestive health. Himalayan pink salt restores electrolytes lost during the night and enhances flavor naturally. Olive oil and lemon zest boost nutrient absorption and add healthy fats. This comforting bowl keeps you full, nourished, and balanced.

CHAPTER 6

Dinner Recipes

Pink Salt-Crusted Lemon Chicken

Preparation Time: 10 minutes   **Cooking Time:** 25 minutes   **Servings:** 2

INGREDIENTS

- Boneless, skinless chicken breasts (2 × 6 oz)
- Himalayan pink salt (½ tsp)
- Black pepper (¼ tsp, freshly ground)
- Garlic powder (½ tsp)
- Lemon zest (1 tsp, finely grated)
- Lemon juice (2 tbsp, freshly squeezed)
- Olive oil (1 tbsp)
- Fresh thyme leaves (1 tsp, chopped)
- Chicken broth (¼ cup, low-sodium)

PREPARATION

1. Preheat oven to 400°F and line a baking dish with parchment paper.
2. Pat chicken breasts dry and place on a cutting board; using a sharp knife, lightly score each breast surface to help seasoning adhere.
3. In a small bowl, combine ½ tsp pink salt, ¼ tsp black pepper, ½ tsp garlic powder, and 1 tsp lemon zest. Rub the mixture evenly onto both sides of each chicken breast.
4. Heat 1 tbsp olive oil in a large ovenproof skillet over medium-high heat; add seasoned chicken and sear 2 minutes per side until golden brown.
5. Pour 2 tbsp lemon juice and ¼ cup chicken broth into the skillet around the chicken, then sprinkle 1 tsp chopped thyme over the breasts.
6. Transfer skillet to the preheated oven and bake 18–20 minutes, or until internal temperature reaches 165°F.
7. Remove chicken from oven and let rest in the skillet for 5 minutes, spooning pan juices over the top before serving.

Benefits: This dish combines lean protein from chicken with electrolytes and trace minerals from pink salt, supporting muscle repair and fluid balance. Lemon zest and juice provide vitamin C and aid in mineral absorption, while thyme offers antioxidants and anti-inflammatory compounds. The gentle pan sear and bake method preserves moisture, ensuring tender, flavorful chicken that promotes satiety and steady energy levels, making it ideal for a balanced dinner.

Baked Cod with Pink Salt & Herbs

Preparation Time: 10 minutes   **Cooking Time:** 15 minutes   **Servings:** 2

INGREDIENTS

- Cod fillets (2 × 6 oz)
- Himalayan pink salt (½ tsp)
- Black pepper (¼ tsp, freshly ground)
- Olive oil (1 tbsp)
- Garlic (1 clove, minced)
- Fresh parsley (2 tbsp, chopped)
- Fresh dill (1 tbsp, chopped)
- Lemon wedges (2, for serving)

PREPARATION

1. Preheat oven to 425°F and line a baking sheet with parchment paper.
2. Pat 2 cod fillets dry and place on the prepared sheet.
3. Drizzle each fillet with ½ tbsp olive oil, then season evenly with ¼ tsp pink salt and ⅛ tsp black pepper per fillet.
4. In a small bowl, combine minced garlic, 2 tbsp parsley, and 1 tbsp dill; sprinkle herb mixture over cod.
5. Bake for 12–15 minutes until fish flakes easily and appears opaque.
6. Serve immediately with lemon wedges for squeezing over the top.

Benefits: Cod provides lean, easily digestible protein and omega-3 fatty acids for heart and brain health. Himalayan pink salt replenishes trace minerals, supporting fluid balance and nerve function. Fresh herbs contribute antioxidants and anti-inflammatory compounds, while lemon adds vitamin C to aid collagen production and iron absorption. This light yet satisfying meal supports muscle recovery and overall wellness.

Pink Salt Pork Tenderloin with Slaw

Preparation Time: 15 minutes | **Cooking Time:** 25 minutes | **Servings:** 2

INGREDIENTS

- Pork tenderloin (12 oz)
- Himalayan pink salt (½ tsp)
- Black pepper (¼ tsp)
- Paprika (½ tsp)
- Olive oil (1 tbsp)
- Green cabbage (1 cup, shredded)
- Carrot (½ cup, shredded)
- Apple cider vinegar (1 tbsp)
- Greek yogurt (1 tbsp)
- Honey (1 tsp)
- Fresh chives (1 tbsp, chopped)

PREPARATION

1. Preheat oven to 400°F. Rub tenderloin with ½ tbsp olive oil, ½ tsp pink salt, ¼ tsp pepper, and ½ tsp paprika.
2. Heat remaining ½ tbsp oil in ovenproof skillet over medium-high heat; sear tenderloin 2 minutes per side until golden.
3. Transfer skillet to oven; roast 20–22 minutes until internal temperature reaches 145°F. Remove and rest 5 minutes.
4. Meanwhile, combine cabbage, carrot, 1 tbsp vinegar, 1 tbsp yogurt, 1 tsp honey, and ½ tsp pink salt in a bowl; toss with chives.
5. Slice pork into ½-inch medallions and serve alongside slaw.

Benefits: Pork tenderloin offers high-quality protein and B vitamins to support energy metabolism. Pink salt restores minerals lost through activity and enhances flavor. The slaw delivers fiber, probiotics from yogurt, and phytonutrients from cabbage and carrots, aiding digestion and immune health. A balanced dish that keeps you full and nourished at dinner.

Cauliflower Rice Stir-Fry with Pink Salt

Preparation Time: 10 minutes | **Cooking Time:** 10 minutes | **Servings:** 2

INGREDIENTS

- Cauliflower (1 medium head, riced, about 3 cups)
- Olive oil (1 tbsp)
- Garlic (2 cloves, minced)
- Carrot (½ cup, diced)
- Peas (½ cup, frozen)
- Himalayan pink salt (½ tsp)
- Tamari or soy sauce (1 tbsp, low-sodium)
- Sesame oil (1 tsp)
- Green onions (2, sliced)
- Sesame seeds (1 tsp, for garnish)

PREPARATION

1. Heat 1 tbsp olive oil in a large skillet over medium heat; sauté garlic 1 minute.
2. Add diced carrot and cook 2–3 minutes until slightly tender.
3. Stir in 3 cups cauliflower rice, ½ cup peas, ½ tsp pink salt, and cook 4 minutes, stirring frequently.
4. Pour 1 tbsp tamari and 1 tsp sesame oil over the mixture; toss to coat.
5. Remove from heat, sprinkle sliced green onions and 1 tsp sesame seeds.

Benefits: This stir-fry swaps grains for cauliflower to lower carbs while boosting vitamin C and fiber. Pink salt supports electrolyte balance. Peas and carrots add plant protein, vitamins, and antioxidants for eye and immune health. Sesame oil and seeds provide healthy fats. A quick, nutrient-dense dinner that keeps you satiated and supports weight-loss goals.

Pink Salt Beef & Broccoli Bowls

Preparation Time: 10 minutes   **Cooking Time:** 15 minutes   **Servings:** 2

INGREDIENTS

- Flank steak (8 oz, thinly sliced)
- Broccoli florets (2 cups)
- Olive oil (1 tbsp)
- Garlic (2 cloves, minced)
- Ginger (1 tsp, grated)
- Himalayan pink salt (½ tsp)
- Black pepper (¼ tsp)
- Low-sodium soy sauce (2 tbsp)
- Rice vinegar (1 tsp)
- Cooked brown rice (2 cups)
- Green onions (2, sliced)

PREPARATION

1. Heat ½ tbsp olive oil in a skillet over medium-high heat; cook steak slices with ¼ tsp pink salt and pepper 2–3 minutes until browned. Transfer to a plate.
2. Add remaining ½ tbsp oil; sauté garlic and ginger 30 seconds.
3. Stir in broccoli and 2 tbsp soy sauce, cover, and cook 4 minutes until crisp-tender.
4. Return steak to skillet, add 1 tsp vinegar and ¼ tsp pink salt, toss to combine and heat through.
5. Divide 2 cups rice between bowls; top with beef and broccoli mixture and garnish with green onions.

Benefits: Lean beef supplies iron and B12 for energy, while broccoli delivers fiber and vitamin K for bone health. Pink salt restores essential minerals. Soy sauce and vinegar add umami for satisfaction without excess sodium. Combined over whole-grain rice, this bowl supports muscle maintenance, stable blood sugar, and digestive health.

Zesty Pink Salt Shrimp Tacos

Preparation Time: 15 minutes   **Cooking Time:** 8 minutes   **Servings:** 4 tacos

INGREDIENTS

- Shrimp (12 large, peeled and deveined)
- Himalayan pink salt (½ tsp)
- Black pepper (¼ tsp)
- Cumin (½ tsp)
- Smoked paprika (½ tsp)
- Olive oil (1 tbsp)
- Corn tortillas (4 small)
- Purple cabbage (1 cup, shredded)
- Avocado (½ medium, sliced)
- Lime wedges (2, for serving)
- Cilantro (2 tbsp, chopped)

PREPARATION

1. In a bowl, toss shrimp with ½ tsp pink salt, ¼ tsp pepper, ½ tsp cumin, and ½ tsp paprika.
2. Heat 1 tbsp olive oil in a skillet over medium-high heat; cook shrimp 2–3 minutes per side until pink and opaque.
3. Warm tortillas in a dry skillet 30 seconds per side.
4. Assemble tacos by layering shredded cabbage, 3 shrimp each, and avocado slices.
5. Garnish with cilantro and serve with lime wedges.

Benefits: Shrimp provide low-calorie protein and selenium for immune support. Pink salt adds trace minerals to aid hydration. Cabbage offers fiber and vitamin C to support digestion and immunity. Corn tortillas keep carbs moderate. The spices enhance metabolism and flavor without fat. These tacos are a fun, balanced dinner that fits your healthy-eating plan.

Veggie-Packed Pink Salt Frittata

Preparation Time: 10 minutes   **Cooking Time:** 20 minutes   **Servings:** 4

INGREDIENTS

- Eggs (8 large)
- Himalayan pink salt (½ tsp)
- Black pepper (¼ tsp, freshly ground)
- Olive oil (1 tbsp)
- Onion (½ cup, diced)
- Bell pepper (½ cup, diced)
- Spinach (1 cup, packed)
- Cherry tomatoes (½ cup, halved)
- Mushrooms (½ cup, sliced)
- Feta cheese (¼ cup, crumbled)

PREPARATION

1. Preheat oven to 375°F. In a bowl, whisk 8 eggs with ½ tsp pink salt and ¼ tsp black pepper.
2. Heat 1 tbsp olive oil in an ovenproof skillet over medium heat; sauté ½ cup onion and ½ cup bell pepper for 3–4 minutes until softened.
3. Add 1 cup spinach, ½ cup mushrooms, and ½ cup cherry tomatoes; cook 2 minutes until spinach wilts.
4. Pour the egg mixture evenly over the vegetables; sprinkle ¼ cup feta on top.
5. Transfer skillet to oven and bake 15–18 minutes until eggs are set and lightly golden.
6. Let rest 5 minutes before slicing into wedges and serving.

Benefits: This frittata is rich in protein and healthy fats from eggs and feta, promoting muscle repair and satiety. Himalayan pink salt adds essential minerals for hydration and nerve function. A variety of vegetables supplies fiber, vitamins, and antioxidants to support digestion and immune health. Quick to make and versatile, it keeps you full and energized for evening activities.

Pink Salt Turkey Meatballs & Zoodles

Preparation Time: 15 minutes   **Cooking Time:** 15 minutes   **Servings:** 2

INGREDIENTS

- Lean ground turkey (8 oz)
- Himalayan pink salt (½ tsp)
- Black pepper (¼ tsp)
- Garlic (1 clove, minced)
- Onion powder (½ tsp)
- Egg (1 large, beaten)
- Parmesan cheese (2 tbsp, grated)
- Olive oil (1 tbsp)
- Zucchini (2 medium, spiralized)
- Cherry tomatoes (½ cup, halved)

PREPARATION

1. In a bowl, combine 8 oz turkey, ½ tsp pink salt, ¼ tsp pepper, 1 minced garlic clove, ½ tsp onion powder, 1 beaten egg, and 2 tbsp Parmesan. Mix gently.
2. Shape mixture into 10 meatballs and set aside.
3. Heat 1 tbsp olive oil in a skillet over medium heat; cook meatballs 6–8 minutes, turning occasionally until browned and cooked through.
4. Remove meatballs; add spiralized zucchini and ½ cup cherry tomatoes to the skillet. Season with a pinch of pink salt and cook 2–3 minutes until tender.
5. Return meatballs to the pan, toss gently with zoodles and tomatoes, then serve immediately.

Benefits: These meatballs provide lean protein to support muscle and recovery, while pink salt ensures electrolyte balance. Zoodles offer a low-carb source of hydration and fiber. Cherry tomatoes add antioxidants and vitamin C, promoting immune health. Parmesan contributes calcium for bone strength. A balanced, flavorful dinner that aligns with weight-loss and wellness goals.

Roasted Veggie & Pink Salt Grain Bowl

Preparation Time: 15 minutes   **Cooking Time:** 30 minutes   **Servings:** 2

INGREDIENTS

- Mixed vegetables (4 cups, e.g., broccoli, cauliflower, carrots)
- Olive oil (2 tbsp)
- Himalayan pink salt (½ tsp)
- Black pepper (to taste)
- Cooked farro or brown rice (2 cups)
- Avocado (1 medium, sliced)
- Tahini dressing (2 tbsp)
- Pumpkin seeds (2 tbsp)

PREPARATION

1. Preheat oven to 425°F and toss 4 cups mixed vegetables with 2 tbsp olive oil, ½ tsp pink salt, and pepper.
2. Roast on a baking sheet 25–30 minutes until tender and golden, stirring halfway through.
3. Divide 2 cups cooked grain between two bowls.
4. Top each bowl with roasted vegetables and sliced avocado.
5. Drizzle 1 tbsp tahini dressing per bowl and sprinkle 1 tbsp pumpkin seeds on top.

Benefits: This bowl combines whole grains for sustained energy with roasted vegetables rich in fiber and micronutrients. Pink salt provides trace minerals vital for hydration. Avocado adds healthy fats for nutrient absorption, and pumpkin seeds offer plant protein and magnesium to support muscle function. A nourishing, balanced meal that fuels recovery and satiety.

Pink Salt-Seasoned Eggplant Parmesan

Preparation Time: 15 minutes   **Cooking Time:** 30 minutes   **Servings:** 2

INGREDIENTS

- Eggplant (1 medium, sliced into ½-inch rounds)
- Himalayan pink salt (½ tsp)
- Black pepper (¼ tsp)
- Olive oil (2 tbsp)
- Marinara sauce (1 cup)
- Mozzarella cheese (½ cup, shredded)
- Parmesan cheese (2 tbsp, grated)
- Fresh basil (2 tbsp, chopped)

PREPARATION

1. Preheat oven to 400°F. Lay eggplant slices on a baking sheet, drizzle with 1 tbsp olive oil, and season with ¼ tsp pink salt and pepper.
2. Roast eggplant 15 minutes, flip slices, then roast another 10 minutes until tender.
3. Reduce oven to 375°F. In a baking dish, layer half the eggplant, ½ cup marinara, ¼ cup mozzarella, and 1 tbsp Parmesan.
4. Repeat layers with remaining eggplant, sauce, and cheeses; sprinkle remaining ¼ tsp salt.
5. Bake 10–12 minutes until cheese melts and bubbles. Garnish with basil before serving.

Benefits: Eggplant delivers fiber and antioxidants like nasunin to protect cells. Pink salt adds mineral support and flavor. Cheese supplies protein and calcium for bone health, while marinara brings lycopene for cardiovascular benefits. A satisfying, vegetable-forward dinner that supports digestion and nutrient balance.

Citrus-Pink Salt Grilled Veggie Skewers

Preparation Time: 15 minutes   **Cooking Time:** 10 minutes   **Servings:** 2

INGREDIENTS

- Zucchini (1 medium, sliced into rounds)
- Red bell pepper (1 medium, cut into squares)
- Red onion (½ medium, cut into wedges)
- Cherry tomatoes (12)
- Olive oil (2 tbsp)
- Himalayan pink salt (½ tsp)
- Black pepper (¼ tsp)
- Lemon zest (1 tsp)
- Lime juice (1 tbsp)
- Wooden skewers (4, soaked if needed)

PREPARATION

1. Toss zucchini, pepper, onion, and tomatoes with 2 tbsp olive oil, ½ tsp pink salt, ¼ tsp pepper, 1 tsp lemon zest, and 1 tbsp lime juice.
2. Thread vegetables onto 4 skewers, alternating colors.
3. Preheat grill or grill pan over medium-high heat; grill skewers 3–4 minutes per side until charred and tender.
4. Transfer to a plate and serve hot, spooning any pan juices over the top.

Benefits: These skewers offer a rainbow of vitamins, minerals, and antioxidants from diverse vegetables. Pink salt restores electrolytes and enhances flavor, while citrus adds vitamin C for immune support. Grilling concentrates natural sugars and adds charred complexity without extra calories. A light, visually appealing dinner for wellness and satiety.

Pink Salt–Infused Cauliflower Steaks

Preparation Time: 10 minutes   **Cooking Time:** 25 minutes   **Servings:** 2

INGREDIENTS

- Cauliflower (1 large head)
- Olive oil (2 tbsp)
- Himalayan pink salt (½ tsp)
- Black pepper (¼ tsp, freshly ground)
- Garlic powder (½ tsp)
- Paprika (½ tsp)
- Fresh parsley (1 tbsp, chopped)
- Lemon wedges (2, for serving)

PREPARATION

1. Preheat oven to 425°F and line a baking sheet with parchment paper.
2. Remove outer leaves from cauliflower and trim stem so head sits flat. Cut into two ¾-inch "steaks." Reserve any loose florets.
3. In a bowl, mix 2 tbsp olive oil, ½ tsp pink salt, ¼ tsp pepper, ½ tsp garlic powder, and ½ tsp paprika.
4. Brush both sides of each steak and reserved florets with the oil-spice blend.
5. Arrange steaks and florets on the sheet without overlapping. Roast 20–25 minutes, flipping halfway, until golden and tender.
6. Transfer to a platter, sprinkle 1 tbsp parsley, and serve with lemon wedges.

Benefits: Cauliflower offers fiber and vitamins C and K for immune and bone health. Pink salt replenishes essential minerals and enhances the vegetable's natural sweetness. Roasting brings out complex flavors without added calories. A nutrient-rich, low-carb entrée that supports digestion, hydration, and metabolic balance.

Wild Rice & Pink Salt Chicken Bake

Preparation Time: 15 minutes   **Cooking Time:** 45 minutes   **Servings:** 4

INGREDIENTS

- Boneless, skinless chicken thighs (4 × 4 oz)
- Wild rice blend (1 cup, rinsed)
- Chicken broth (2½ cups, low-sodium)
- Himalayan pink salt (1 tsp, divided)
- Black pepper (¼ tsp)
- Olive oil (1 tbsp)
- Onion (1 cup, diced)
- Mushrooms (1 cup, sliced)
- Carrot (1 cup, sliced)
- Thyme (1 tbsp, fresh leaves)

PREPARATION

1. Preheat oven to 375°F. In a skillet, heat 1 tbsp olive oil over medium heat; sauté 1 cup onion and mushrooms 4 minutes.
2. Stir in 1 cup carrot and cook 2 minutes. Season with ½ tsp pink salt and ¼ tsp pepper.
3. Transfer vegetables to a 9×13-inch baking dish; spread 1 cup wild rice blend evenly.
4. Nestle 4 chicken thighs atop rice. Sprinkle remaining ½ tsp salt and thyme over the chicken.
5. Pour 2½ cups broth into the dish, cover tightly with foil, and bake 40 minutes.
6. Remove foil and bake 5 more minutes to brown the chicken. Let rest 5 minutes before serving.

Benefits: Wild rice offers complex carbohydrates, fiber, and magnesium for energy and digestive health. Chicken thighs provide moist, flavorful protein and iron. Pink salt restores electrolytes, and fresh vegetables supply vitamins and antioxidants. A one-dish meal that supports balanced nutrition, sustained energy, and minimal cleanup, perfect for a wholesome dinner.

Pink Salt Lamb Chops with Mint Sauce

Preparation Time: 10 minutes   **Cooking Time:** 15 minutes   **Servings:** 2

INGREDIENTS

- Lamb chops (4 × 3 oz)
- Himalayan pink salt (½ tsp)
- Black pepper (¼ tsp)
- Olive oil (1 tbsp)
- Fresh mint leaves (¼ cup, packed)
- Greek yogurt (2 tbsp)
- Lemon juice (1 tsp)
- Garlic (1 small clove)
- Green beans (1 cup, trimmed, steamed)

PREPARATION

1. Season lamb chops with ½ tsp pink salt and ¼ tsp pepper on both sides.
2. Heat 1 tbsp olive oil in a skillet over medium-high heat; cook chops 3–4 minutes per side for medium doneness. Transfer to a plate to rest.
3. In a blender, combine ¼ cup mint, 2 tbsp yogurt, 1 tsp lemon juice, and garlic clove; blend until smooth.
4. Steam 1 cup green beans until bright green and tender-crisp.
5. Serve lamb chops topped with mint sauce alongside green beans.

Benefits: Lamb chops deliver high-quality protein, B vitamins, and zinc for immune support and muscle maintenance. Pink salt restores trace minerals and enhances savory flavor. Mint sauce adds digestive benefits and antioxidants, while yogurt provides probiotics. Green beans supply fiber and vitamin K for bone health. A gourmet-style dinner that nourishes and delights.

Creamy Avocado & Pink Salt Pasta

Preparation Time: 10 minutes   **Cooking Time:** 12 minutes   **Servings:** 2

INGREDIENTS

- Whole-grain pasta (4 oz)
- Avocado (1 medium, ripe)
- Himalayan pink salt (½ tsp)
- Garlic (1 clove)
- Lemon juice (1 tbsp)
- Olive oil (1 tbsp)
- Cherry tomatoes (½ cup, halved)
- Basil (2 tbsp, chopped)
- Red pepper flakes (¼ tsp, optional)

PREPARATION

1. Cook 4 oz pasta according to package instructions until al dente; reserve ¼ cup cooking water and drain.
2. In a blender, combine avocado, ½ tsp pink salt, garlic clove, 1 tbsp lemon juice, 1 tbsp oil, and 2 tbsp reserved water; blend until creamy.
3. Return pasta to the pot over low heat; pour in avocado sauce and toss to coat, adding more cooking water if needed.
4. Stir in cherry tomatoes and basil; heat 1 minute.
5. Divide between plates and sprinkle with red pepper flakes if desired.

Benefits: This pasta combines whole grains for complex carbs and avocado for heart-healthy fats and potassium, aiding fluid balance. Pink salt supplies essential trace minerals. Garlic and lemon boost flavor and immunity, while tomatoes add lycopene. A creamy, plant-based sauce that supports satiety, nutrient absorption, and steady energy for evening activities.

CHAPTER 7

Snack Recipes

Pink Salt & Rosemary Roasted Nuts

Preparation Time: 5 minutes   **Cooking Time:** 15 minutes   **Servings:** 4

INGREDIENTS

- Raw mixed nuts (2 cups; e.g., almonds, cashews, walnuts)
- Olive oil (1 tbsp)
- Himalayan pink salt (½ tsp)
- Fresh rosemary (1 tsp, finely chopped)
- Freshly ground black pepper (¼ tsp)

PREPARATION

1. Preheat oven to 350°F and line a baking sheet with parchment paper.
2. In a large bowl, combine 2 cups raw mixed nuts and 1 tbsp olive oil; toss until nuts are evenly coated.
3. Sprinkle ½ tsp pink salt, 1 tsp chopped rosemary, and ¼ tsp black pepper over the oiled nuts; mix thoroughly.
4. Spread the seasoned nuts in a single layer on the prepared baking sheet.
5. Roast for 12–15 minutes, stirring once at the 8-minute mark to ensure even toasting.
6. Remove from oven and let cool on the baking sheet for 5 minutes; transfer to a serving bowl.

Benefits: These roasted nuts offer a convenient source of healthy fats, plant protein, and dietary fiber, helping to stabilize blood sugar and curb mid-afternoon cravings. Pink salt replenishes trace minerals and supports electrolyte balance, while rosemary provides antioxidants and anti-inflammatory compounds that may aid circulation and cognitive function. The mild heat from black pepper enhances nutrient absorption, making this snack both flavorful and nourishing for sustained energy between meals.

Veggie Sticks with Pink Salt Hummus

Preparation Time: 10 minutes **Cooking Time:** 0 minutes **Servings:** 4

INGREDIENTS

- Canned chickpeas (15 oz, drained and rinsed)
- Tahini (2 tbsp)
- Lemon juice (2 tbsp, freshly squeezed)
- Himalayan pink salt (½ tsp)
- Garlic (1 clove, minced)
- Olive oil (1 tbsp, plus extra for drizzling)
- Water (2–3 tbsp, as needed)
- Carrot sticks (1 cup)
- Cucumber sticks (1 cup)
- Bell pepper sticks (1 cup, mixed colors)

PREPARATION

1. In a food processor, combine 15 oz chickpeas, 2 tbsp tahini, 2 tbsp lemon juice, ½ tsp pink salt, and minced garlic.
2. Process while drizzling 1 tbsp olive oil; add 2–3 tbsp water to reach desired creaminess.
3. Transfer hummus to a serving bowl and drizzle with additional olive oil if desired.
4. Arrange carrot, cucumber, and bell pepper sticks on a platter alongside the hummus.
5. Sprinkle a small pinch (a few grains) of pink salt over the top of the hummus for garnish.

Benefits: This snack combines fiber and plant protein from chickpeas and vegetables to support digestive health and maintain steady energy. Pink salt adds trace minerals that aid hydration and muscle function. Tahini contributes healthy fats and calcium, while fresh veggies deliver vitamins and phytonutrients for immune support. The creamy hummus paired with crisp veggie sticks makes for a satisfying, nutrient-rich snack that curbs cravings.

Pink Salt–Sprinkled Kale Chips

Preparation Time: 5 minutes **Cooking Time:** 15 minutes **Servings:** 3

INGREDIENTS

- Curly kale leaves (6 cups, stems removed, torn into bite-size)
- Olive oil (1 tbsp)
- Himalayan pink salt (¼ tsp)
- Black pepper (to taste)

PREPARATION

1. Preheat oven to 300°F and line a baking sheet with parchment paper.
2. In a large bowl, toss kale leaves with 1 tbsp olive oil until evenly coated.
3. Spread kale in a single layer on the baking sheet; sprinkle ¼ tsp pink salt and pepper.
4. Bake for 12–15 minutes until kale is crisp but not browned, rotating the pan halfway through.
5. Remove and let cool slightly; transfer to a serving bowl.

Benefits: Kale chips deliver concentrated vitamins A, C, and K, along with fiber to support gut health. Pink salt provides essential trace minerals for hydration and nerve function. The baking method preserves nutrients while achieving a satisfying crunch without added starch or empty calories. A light, nutrient-packed snack that helps maintain energy and supports overall wellness.

Energy Bites with Pink Salt & Dates

Preparation Time: 10 minutes   **Cooking Time:** 0 minutes   **Servings:** 12 bites

INGREDIENTS

- Pitted Medjool dates (1 cup)
- Old-fashioned oats (1 cup)
- Almond butter (½ cup)
- Himalayan pink salt (¼ tsp)
- Chia seeds (2 tbsp)
- Vanilla extract (1 tsp)
- Shredded coconut (2 tbsp, for rolling)

PREPARATION

1. In a food processor, pulse 1 cup dates until they form a paste.
2. Add 1 cup oats, ½ cup almond butter, 2 tbsp chia seeds, ¼ tsp pink salt, and 1 tsp vanilla; process until mixture sticks together.
3. Scoop 1 tbsp portions and roll into balls.
4. Roll each ball in 2 tbsp shredded coconut to coat.
5. Refrigerate bites for 30 minutes before serving.

Benefits: These energy bites combine natural sugars from dates for quick fuel with oats and chia seeds for sustained energy release. Pink salt restores electrolytes, and almond butter supplies healthy fats and protein to curb hunger. Coconut adds texture and medium-chain triglycerides for metabolism support. An easy, portable snack perfect for pre- or mid-workout boosts.

Pink Salt Dark Chocolate Bark

Preparation Time: 5 minutes   **Cooking Time:** 10 minutes (setting time)   **Servings:** 8 pieces

INGREDIENTS

- Dark chocolate (6 oz, 70% cacao minimum)
- Himalayan pink salt (½ tsp, coarse)
- Almonds (2 tbsp, chopped)
- Dried cranberries (2 tbsp)

PREPARATION

1. Line a baking sheet with parchment paper.
2. Melt 6 oz chocolate in a heatproof bowl over simmering water, stirring until smooth.
3. Pour melted chocolate onto parchment and spread to ¼-inch thickness.
4. Sprinkle 2 tbsp chopped almonds, 2 tbsp cranberries, and ½ tsp pink salt evenly over the surface.
5. Refrigerate 10 minutes until set; break into 8 pieces.

Benefits: Dark chocolate delivers antioxidants like flavonoids that support heart health and mood. Pink salt adds essential minerals and heightens flavor. Nuts contribute healthy fats and protein, while cranberries offer vitamin C and fiber. A rich yet balanced treat that satisfies sweet cravings while providing nutritional benefits.

Citrus-Pink Salt Fruit Salad Cups

Preparation Time: 10 minutes   **Cooking Time:** 0 minutes   **Servings:** 4

INGREDIENTS

- Orange (1 large, segmented)
- Grapefruit (1 medium, segmented)
- Pineapple (1 cup, diced)
- Kiwi (2, peeled and sliced)
- Himalayan pink salt (¼ tsp)
- Honey (1 tsp, optional)
- Mint leaves (4, for garnish)

PREPARATION

1. In a large bowl, combine orange segments, grapefruit segments, pineapple, and kiwi slices.
2. Drizzle 1 tsp honey if desired, then sprinkle ¼ tsp pink salt over the fruit.
3. Gently toss to distribute salt and honey.
4. Divide salad into 4 cups and garnish each with a mint leaf.

Benefits: This fruit salad combines hydrating citrus and pineapple rich in vitamin C and digestive enzymes. Pink salt restores minerals and enhances natural sweetness. Kiwi adds fiber and antioxidants. A refreshing, nutrient-dense snack that supports hydration, digestion, and immune health, ideal for any time of day.

Pink Salt Seaweed Crisps

Preparation Time: 5 minutes   **Cooking Time:** 10 minutes   **Servings:** 4

INGREDIENTS

- Roasted seaweed sheets (4, full-size)
- Sesame oil (1 tsp)
- Himalayan pink salt (¼ tsp, finely ground)

PREPARATION

1. Preheat oven to 275°F and line a baking sheet with parchment paper.
2. Lightly brush both sides of each seaweed sheet with 1 tsp sesame oil.
3. Stack sheets and cut into quarters.
4. Arrange crisps in a single layer on the sheet and sprinkle evenly with ¼ tsp pink salt.
5. Bake 8–10 minutes until crisp but not browned; remove and let cool.

Benefits: Seaweed offers iodine and trace minerals essential for thyroid and metabolic health. Pink salt adds electrolytes that complement seaweed's mineral profile. Sesame oil provides healthy fats and a toasty note. These crisps deliver a low-calorie, nutrient-dense snack that supports hydration, energy production, and balanced electrolytes.

Greek Yogurt Dip with Pink Salt Herbs

Preparation Time: 10 minutes   **Cooking Time:** 0 minutes   **Servings:** 4

INGREDIENTS

- Greek yogurt (1 cup, plain)
- Himalayan pink salt (½ tsp)
- Black pepper (to taste)
- Fresh dill (1 tbsp, chopped)
- Fresh chives (1 tbsp, chopped)
- Lemon juice (1 tsp, freshly squeezed)
- Garlic powder (¼ tsp)

PREPARATION

1. In a bowl, stir together 1 cup yogurt, ½ tsp pink salt, and ¼ tsp garlic powder.
2. Add chopped dill, chives, and 1 tsp lemon juice; mix until uniform.
3. Season with pepper to taste.
4. Chill 10 minutes to meld flavors, then serve with fresh veggies or crackers.

Benefits: This dip provides probiotics for gut health, protein for satiety, and trace minerals for electrolyte balance from pink salt. Fresh herbs add antioxidants and flavor without calories, while lemon juice aids digestion. A versatile, creamy snack that supports digestion, immune function, and sustained energy.

Pink Salt–Seasoned Edamame

Preparation Time: 5 minutes   **Cooking Time:** 5 minutes   **Servings:** 2

INGREDIENTS

- Frozen edamame in pods (1 cup)
- Himalayan pink salt (½ tsp)
- Black pepper (¼ tsp)
- Olive oil (1 tsp)

PREPARATION

1. Bring a small pot of water to a boil; add edamame and cook 4 minutes.
2. Drain and transfer pods to a bowl; drizzle with 1 tsp olive oil.
3. Sprinkle ½ tsp pink salt and ¼ tsp pepper; toss to coat.
4. Serve warm, squeezing pods to pop beans into mouth.

Benefits: Edamame delivers complete plant protein, fiber, and folate to support muscle repair and digestion. Pink salt adds essential minerals, while olive oil supplies healthy fats. A quick, satisfying snack that stabilizes blood sugar, hydrates, and supports metabolic function.

Apple Slices with Pink Salt Almond Butter

Preparation Time: 5 minutes   **Cooking Time:** 0 minutes   **Servings:** 2

INGREDIENTS

- Apple (1 medium, cored and sliced)
- Almond butter (2 tbsp)
- Himalayan pink salt (⅛ tsp)
- Ground cinnamon (¼ tsp, optional)

PREPARATION

1. Arrange sliced apple on a plate.
2. Spread 1 tbsp almond butter on each apple slice, or offer it for dipping.
3. Sprinkle ⅛ tsp pink salt evenly over the almond butter.
4. Dust with ¼ tsp cinnamon if using, and serve.

Benefits: This snack balances natural fruit sugars with protein and healthy fats to curb cravings and stabilize blood sugar. Pink salt replenishes electrolytes. Almond butter provides vitamin E and magnesium for muscle and nerve function. Apples deliver fiber and antioxidants, supporting digestion and immune health. A simple, nutrient-rich treat.

Pink Salt & Lemon Protein Bars

Preparation Time: 15 minutes   **Cooking Time:** 10 minutes   **Servings:** 8 bars

INGREDIENTS

- Rolled oats (1 cup)
- Protein powder (½ cup, vanilla)
- Almond flour (¼ cup)
- Honey (½ cup)
- Almond butter (¼ cup)
- Lemon zest (1 tbsp)
- Lemon juice (2 tbsp)
- Himalayan pink salt (½ tsp)
- Chia seeds (2 tbsp)

PREPARATION

1. Preheat oven to 350°F and line an 8×8-inch pan with parchment.
2. In a bowl, combine 1 cup oats, ½ cup protein powder, ¼ cup almond flour, 2 tbsp chia, and ½ tsp salt.
3. Gently heat ½ cup honey and ¼ cup almond butter until pourable; stir in zest and juice.
4. Pour wet into dry ingredients; mix until uniform.
5. Press mixture into pan and bake 10 minutes. Let cool fully, then cut into 8 bars.

Benefits: These bars provide balanced macronutrients—protein for muscle repair, healthy fats for satiety, and oats for fiber. Pink salt replenishes minerals lost through activity. Lemon adds vitamin C and a refreshing flavor. Chia seeds contribute omega-3s and hydration support. A portable, energizing snack ideal for workouts or busy afternoons.

Cucumber Rounds with Pink Salt Tzatziki

Preparation Time: 10 minutes   **Cooking Time:** 0 minutes   **Servings:** 4

INGREDIENTS

- Cucumber (1 large, sliced into ½-inch rounds)
- Greek yogurt (½ cup, plain)
- Himalayan pink salt (¼ tsp)
- Fresh dill (1 tbsp, chopped)
- Garlic (½ clove, minced)
- Lemon juice (1 tsp, freshly squeezed)
- Olive oil (1 tsp)

PREPARATION

1. In a small bowl, combine ½ cup Greek yogurt, ¼ tsp pink salt, ½ clove minced garlic, 1 tbsp dill, and 1 tsp lemon juice; stir until smooth.
2. Drizzle 1 tsp olive oil into the tzatziki and mix gently.
3. Arrange cucumber rounds on a serving plate.
4. Top each slice with a dollop (about 1 tsp) of tzatziki.
5. Garnish with a small sprig of dill and serve.

Benefits: Crisp cucumber provides hydration and fiber, aiding digestion and refreshment. The yogurt-based tzatziki delivers probiotics for gut health and protein for satiety. Pink salt replenishes trace minerals and enhances flavor. Garlic and dill add antioxidants and anti-inflammatory properties. Together, this snack balances hydration, digestion support, and sustained energy in a light, flavorful bite.

Pink Salt–Roasted Chickpeas

Preparation Time: 5 minutes   **Cooking Time:** 30 minutes   **Servings:** 4

INGREDIENTS

- Canned chickpeas (15 oz, drained, rinsed, patted dry)
- Olive oil (1 tbsp)
- Himalayan pink salt (½ tsp)
- Paprika (½ tsp)
- Ground cumin (¼ tsp)
- Black pepper (to taste)

PREPARATION

1. Preheat oven to 400°F and line a baking sheet with parchment paper.
2. Toss chickpeas with 1 tbsp olive oil, ensuring an even coat.
3. Sprinkle ½ tsp pink salt, ½ tsp paprika, ¼ tsp cumin, and pepper; stir to distribute spices.
4. Spread chickpeas in a single layer on the sheet.
5. Roast 25–30 minutes, shaking the pan every 10 minutes, until golden and crisp.
6. Cool slightly before serving.

Benefits: Chickpeas offer plant-based protein and fiber to support blood sugar balance and digestive health. Pink salt provides essential minerals for hydration and nerve function. The spices add antioxidants and depth of flavor without excess calories. This crunchy snack delivers sustained energy and satisfies savory cravings.

Mini Pink Salt Quiches

Preparation Time: 10 minutes   **Cooking Time:** 20 minutes   **Servings:** 6 mini quiches

INGREDIENTS

- Eggs (3 large)
- Milk (¼ cup, any variety)
- Himalayan pink salt (¼ tsp)
- Black pepper (to taste)
- Pre-made pie crust (1 sheet, cut into 6 rounds)
- Cheddar cheese (¼ cup, shredded)
- Spinach (¼ cup, chopped)
- Red bell pepper (2 tbsp, diced)

PREPARATION

1. Preheat oven to 375°F and grease a 6-cup muffin tin.
2. Press pie crust rounds into each cup.
3. In a bowl, whisk 3 eggs, ¼ cup milk, ¼ tsp pink salt, and pepper.
4. Divide ¼ cup cheese, ¼ cup spinach, and 2 tbsp bell pepper among crust-lined cups.
5. Pour egg mixture evenly into each until just below the rim.
6. Bake 18–20 minutes until set and golden. Let cool 5 minutes before removing.

Benefits: These mini quiches pack protein and healthy fats from eggs and cheese, stabilizing blood sugar and supporting muscle recovery. Pink salt adds vital trace minerals. Vegetables contribute fiber, vitamins, and antioxidants for immune and digestive health. Bite-size portions make them perfect for portion control and on-the-go nourishment.

Pink Salt Popcorn with Nutritional Yeast

Preparation Time: 5 minutes   **Cooking Time:** 5 minutes   **Servings:** 2

INGREDIENTS

- Popcorn kernels (½ cup)
- Olive oil (1 tbsp)
- Himalayan pink salt (¼ tsp)
- Nutritional yeast (2 tbsp)

PREPARATION

1. Heat 1 tbsp oil in a large pot over medium heat; add ½ cup kernels and cover.
2. Shake pot occasionally until popping slows (about 2 seconds between pops); remove from heat.
3. Transfer popcorn to a large bowl.
4. Sprinkle ¼ tsp pink salt and 2 tbsp nutritional yeast; toss to coat evenly.

Benefits: Popcorn is a whole-grain, low-calorie source of fiber for digestive health. Nutritional yeast adds B vitamins and a savory, cheesy flavor without dairy. Pink salt replenishes electrolytes and enhances taste. This snack provides satisfying crunch and nutrients that support energy metabolism and gut function.

CHAPTER 8

Troubleshooting & FAQs

NAVIGATING COMMON PLATEAUS

Hitting a plateau can feel like running on a treadmill: you're working hard but not moving forward. During a 21-day pink salt ritual, progress often shows up in the first two weeks—weight shifts, more energy, clearer digestion. Around day 14 or 15, however, many people find that changes slow or stall. Understanding why plateaus occur and learning how to move past them can make the difference between frustration and long-term success.

Plateaus happen for several reasons. Your body adapts to a new routine—metabolism may adjust to the calorie intake and activity level you established. Hormones like insulin and cortisol can reset their responses, slowing fat burning. Water retention fluctuates based on sodium balance, stress, and carbohydrates. Even small changes in sleep or daily stress can affect hormones and digestion, masking fat loss. Recognizing these shifts as normal rather than failures helps you stay motivated.

Recognizing a Plateau

First, you need to know you're on one. If your weight, measurements, or energy levels haven't budged for three consecutive days, you may be in a plateau phase. Relying on the scale alone can be misleading—fluctuations of one to two pounds of water weight are common. Instead, track multiple markers:

- Daily weight at the same time—ideally first thing in the morning after restroom use and before eating.
- Weekly measurements of waist, hips, and chest to gauge inches lost.
- Energy logs noting how you feel two hours after your pink salt elixir and mid-day energy peaks or slumps.
- Subjective markers such as mood, hunger, and sleep quality recorded in your journal.

When several of these indicators flatten out, you've likely hit a plateau. Rather than pushing harder immediately, take a moment to review your routine and habits.

Strategies to Overcome Plateaus

Once you spot a plateau, you can adjust three main levers: nutrition, movement, and ritual timing.

Nutrition Tweaks

Your pink salt ritual contributes electrolytes and gentle hydration but calories from meals and snacks drive energy balance. To shake things up:

- Reduce refined carbs slightly—swap white rice, bread, or pasta for more vegetables or a small portion of high-fiber grains like barley.
- Cycle your caloric intake—eat 200 to 300 extra calories on one active day per week, then return to your normal intake to prevent metabolic slow-down.
- Increase protein by 5 to 10 grams per meal to boost satiety and support muscle mass, which in turn burns more calories at rest.

These changes prompt your body to re-evaluate fuel needs and can kick-start additional fat burning without drastic dieting.

Movement Adjustments

If you've been consistent with the same walks, workouts, or yoga flows for two weeks, your muscles have adapted. To spark new calorie burn:

- Add one interval session per week—alternating 30 seconds of brisk effort (fast walking, jogging, cycling) with 60 seconds of recovery for 10–15 minutes.
- Incorporate resistance moves—body-weight squats, push-ups, or dumbbell rows two days a week to build lean tissue.
- Change your environment—move outdoors, try a different class, or explore a new trail to challenge coordination and engage different muscle groups.

These variations force your body to use energy in unfamiliar ways, elevating post-exercise calorie burn and preventing stagnation.

Ritual Timing and Add-Ins

Even your pink salt protocol can adapt. If you've been taking your elixir only in the morning, consider:

- Adding a second glass mid-afternoon to sustain hydration and curb energy dips.
- Pairing the elixir with a breath-movement mini-sequence—two minutes of box breathing and hip circles—to boost circulation and stimulate metabolism twice daily.
- Experimenting with flavor add-ins like a pinch of cinnamon or a splash of apple cider vinegar to engage different digestive responses.

These small shifts keep your ritual fresh and your body guessing, helping to overcome adaptive responses.

Case Example: Breaking Through Week Three

Consider Maria, a marketing executive juggling deadlines and family life. She began the pink salt challenge with daily morning elixirs, three workouts per week, and balanced meals. By day 14, she'd lost five pounds and felt energized. From day 15 to 18, her scale didn't budge, and she felt hungrier. Instead of cutting calories further, she:

1. Added 5 grams of protein powder to her afternoon smoothie.
2. Swapped her evening walk for a 15-minute interval of fast-paced lunges interspersed with resting stands.
3. Sipped a second pink salt elixir at 3 p.m. paired with deep belly breaths.

By day 21, not only did Maria resume gradual weight loss, but she also reported fewer afternoon crashes and a clearer head during late meetings. Her body responded to the adjusted nutrition, movement, and ritual cues.

Embracing Plateaus as Part of Progress

Plateaus can feel like setbacks, but they are simply signals that your body needs variation and attentive care. Tracking multiple markers and employing targeted tweaks in meals, workouts, and your pink salt ritual will help you move past stalls. With each iteration, you learn more about how your unique metabolism responds and how small adjustments can reignite progress and keep you on track toward your goals.

MANAGING SODIUM INTAKE & BALANCE

When you begin incorporating pink salt into your daily routine, you're purposefully adding a source of sodium—an electrolyte that affects fluid balance, nerve signals, and muscle function. Yet, sodium can be both a friend and a foe. Too little may leave you dizzy, fatigued, or prone to muscle cramps; too much can cause bloating, spikes in blood pressure, and headaches. Finding your personal sweet spot requires attention to total sodium intake from all sources—pink salt, packaged foods, cooking salt, and restaurant meals—and matching it to your activity, climate, and health profile.

The Role of Sodium in Your Ritual

Every time you stir pink salt into water, you're tapping into its mineral profile—primarily sodium chloride with trace elements. When you start the morning with your elixir, you give your cells the push they need to rehydrate after eight hours without fluids. Sodium draws water into the bloodstream and cells, supporting circulation and digestion. As you move through your day—especially if you exercise or live in a hot climate—you lose sodium in sweat. Replacing it prevents cramps, maintains energy, and keeps your 21-day challenge on track.

However, most people already get substantial sodium from their regular diet. The average American consumes more than 3,400 mg per day—well above the 2,300 mg upper limit recommended by the Dietary Guidelines for Americans. Add 200–400 mg from your morning pink salt drink, and you may unintentionally cross a threshold that leads to water retention or high blood pressure.

Signs You're Overdoing Sodium

- You feel puffier around your ankles or fingers, especially later in the day.
- Your resting blood pressure reads higher than usual, even after a week of consistent measurement.
- You notice persistent bloating or discomfort in your abdomen.
- You experience frequent headaches or sudden thirst spikes unrelated to exercise.

If any of these sound familiar, adjusting your intake can relieve symptoms and stabilize your progress.

Practical Ways to Balance Sodium

Achieving balance isn't about cutting all salt; it's about matching sodium supply to your personal loss. Here are strategies to help you dial in the right amount:

- Track all sources of sodium, not just your pink salt. Use a nutrition app or food journal to record packaged foods, condiments, and restaurant items.
- Read nutrition labels carefully. A single cup of canned soup may contain 800 mg of sodium—almost half your daily goal—even before you add any pink salt elixir.
- Shift to lower-sodium versions of common staples. Choose reduced-sodium broths, canned beans labeled "no salt added," and breads marked "less sodium."
- Adjust your pink salt dose. If you're already near 2,300 mg daily, consider reducing your morning pinch from ¼ teaspoon to ⅛ teaspoon, or alternate days.
- Swap high-sodium snacks for fresh options. Instead of jerky or chips, reach for fruit cups or raw vegetables paired with low-sodium dips.
- Hydrate proactively. Drinking water throughout the day helps kidneys flush excess sodium and keeps you from confusing thirst with hunger.

By taking inventory of every salty spoonful and reading labels, you'll discover hidden sources that may be pushing you over your comfort zone.

Pairing Sodium with Potassium and Water

Sodium works hand in hand with other electrolytes—potassium, magnesium, and calcium—to regulate fluid and nerve signaling. When you increase sodium, it's wise to up potassium too. Foods rich in potassium—bananas, sweet potatoes, spinach, and avocados—help your body excrete extra sodium and support muscle function. Consider adding a potassium-rich smoothie mid-day or including a side of sautéed greens at dinner.

Water intake is equally important. Even mild dehydration concentrates sodium in your blood, making you crave more fluids and potentially more salt. Aim for at least eight glasses a day, more when you exercise or sweat heavily. If you notice dark-colored urine or dry mouth, you may need to sip more water before reaching for extra salt.

A Case Study: Finding Your Balance

Imagine Sarah, a busy sales manager in Phoenix. She began the pink salt ritual with ¼ teaspoon each morning. During cooler mornings, she felt great: more clarity, fewer muscle aches. But as temperatures climbed above 100°F, she noticed swelling in her ankles and afternoon headaches. Sarah logged her meals and realized she was eating two deli-sandwich lunches per week, each with 900 mg of sodium, plus dressings and pickles. Adding 400 mg from pink salt pushed her to nearly 4,000 mg daily.

- To rebalance, Sarah:
- Swapped deli sandwiches for grilled chicken salads with homemade low-sodium vinaigrette.
- Reduced pink salt to ⅛ teaspoon on weekdays and left it at ¼ teaspoon on heavy workout days.
- Added a potassium smoothie mid-afternoon—spinach, banana, and coconut water.
- Increased her water goal from eight to ten cups daily.

Within a week, her swelling resolved, headaches stopped, and she maintained the energy boost of her morning elixir without setbacks.

Adjusting for Health Conditions

If you have high blood pressure, kidney issues, or heart concerns, sodium management requires extra care. Consult your healthcare provider before starting any new salt-based protocol. They may recommend:

- Monitoring daily blood pressure at home and sharing readings with your provider.
- Lowering total sodium to 1,500 mg per day while using pink salt sparingly or under guidance.
- Pairing your ritual with dietitian-crafted meal plans that accommodate medical needs.

Medical advice ensures that your pink salt ritual supports your health rather than unintentionally complicating it.

Managing sodium isn't about fear of salt; it's about mastering the balance that lets you harness the benefits of pink salt—better hydration, smoother digestion, heightened energy—while avoiding unwanted side effects. By tracking intake, adjusting doses, pairing with potassium and water, and listening to your body, you create a flexible protocol that adapts to your daily life, your climate, and your health history.

OVERCOMING CRAVINGS & ENERGY SLUMPS

When you commit to a 21-day pink salt ritual, you often feel a surge of energy in the first week—mental clarity, steady appetite, fewer mid-afternoon swings. Yet around days 10 to 14, cravings for sweets or salty snacks can creep in, and energy dips might return. These moments aren't failures but signals from your body: hormones, blood sugar, hydration, and nutrient levels are shifting. Learning to decode these cravings and reinvigorate your energy helps you stay on track and feel more in control of your progress.

Recognizing Craving and Slump Triggers

Cravings and slumps arise from a mix of physical factors and habitual patterns. When blood sugar drops, your brain yells for quick fuel—often in the form of refined carbs. Stress raises cortisol, which can trigger hunger even when you've eaten enough. Dehydration, common when increasing pink salt intake without matching fluids, may masquerade as hunger. Skipping meals or following overly strict diets can backfire, causing sudden hunger and fatigue.

- Blood sugar dips after skipping lunch or relying on low-volume salads without balanced macros.
- Emotional triggers such as deadlines, family stress, or worry about hitting goals prompt comfort eating.
- Inadequate hydration—where thirst feels like an "empty" sensation—leads to reaching for snacks.
- Hormonal fluctuations, especially mid-day cortisol peaks, can create both cravings and an inability to focus.

By keeping a simple log—note what you ate, how you felt two hours later, and whether you experienced a craving—you begin to spot patterns. For example, Sarah, a marketing manager, realized her 3 p.m. slump and cookie craving always followed a meeting she found stressful. Recognizing that allowed her to shift her snack strategy.

Nutritional Strategies to Curb Cravings

Balancing carbohydrates, protein, and healthy fats at each meal stabilizes blood sugar and keeps your appetite in check. Your morning pink salt elixir jump-starts hydration and electrolytes, but what you eat afterward matters just as much.

Pair Protein with Every Snack

Protein slows digestion of carbohydrates and provides amino acids that support mood and energy. Instead of a handful of chips, reach for:

- A hard-boiled egg and a few cashews to deliver 8–10 grams of protein and healthy fats.
- A small Greek yogurt parfait with berries and a sprinkle of pink salt for protein, calcium, and antioxidants.
- Turkey-avocado lettuce cups for lean protein, fiber, and minerals that satisfy hunger longer.

When Maria, a busy mom, swapped her 4 p.m. mini chocolate bar for almond-flour waffles paired with cottage cheese, her cravings dropped and she had steady energy until dinner.

Choose Low-Glycemic Carbs

Low-glycemic fruits, whole grains, and vegetables release sugar into the bloodstream slowly, avoiding sudden crashes:

- Half a sweet potato with a pinch of pink salt as a mid-afternoon snack.
- A small bowl of quinoa salad with herbs and lemon to provide sustained fuel and fiber.
- Veggie sticks dipped in protein-rich hummus for crunch plus complex carbohydrates.

These snacks deliver vitamins, minerals, and fiber that support digestion and help you ride out a slump without the roller-coaster of spikes and dips.

Hydration and Electrolytes

Dehydration intensifies both fatigue and cravings. Your pink salt elixir helps replace sodium, but you need adequate water throughout the day:

- Sip water with a slice of cucumber or a squirt of lemon between meals to keep fluid levels optimal.
- When you feel a craving, pause and drink 8 ounces of water, waiting five minutes to see if it subsides.
- Consider herbal teas or infused water—rosehip, ginger, or mint—to add variety without extra sugar.

In one study, even mild dehydration (1–2 percent body weight) impaired mood and concentration. By prioritizing hydration, you lessen the urge to reach for quick fixes.

Ritual and Movement Hacks to Boost Energy

Sometimes cravings appear not because of actual hunger but boredom or stress. Integrating small rituals and movement breaks can reset your focus and reduce emotional eating.

Mini Movement Bursts

Short, targeted movements increase circulation, raise endorphins, and boost metabolism, counteracting afternoon fatigue:

- Two minutes of chair squats or wall-push-ups at your desk to oxygenate muscles and mind.
- A quick walk around the block or stair climb for five minutes to break cognitive fog.
- A brief yoga sequence—cat-cow and child's pose—to relieve tension and reset breathing.

When David, an IT specialist, swapped his chip break at 3 p.m. for a walk around the office, he found his energy rebounded and his urge to snack waned.

Breathing and Mindfulness

Adding a simple breathing or mindfulness pause can curb emotional cravings:

- Practice box breathing—inhale for four counts, hold for four, exhale for four, hold for four—three times when stress spikes.
- A five-minute guided meditation or body scan app session to reduce cortisol and reset appetite cues.
- Take a moment to note three things you're grateful for before reaching for a snack—to differentiate true hunger from habit.

These quick practices create space between urge and action, giving you the chance to choose a healthier option.

Flavor and Texture Substitutes

Often cravings are for a specific mouthfeel—crunch, creaminess, sweetness—rather than nutrition. You can meet that need without derailing progress:

- Crunch: reach for kale chips with a pinch of pink salt instead of potato chips.
- Creamy: swirl yogurt with a teaspoon of nut butter and cinnamon rather than a candy bar.
- Sweet: nibble on a few dates sprinkled with salt instead of slices of cake.

By replicating the sensory experience, you satisfy your palate while staying aligned with your goals.

Tracking your snacks, fluids, and energy levels—then matching them to targeted strategies—lets you overcome cravings and slumps with intention rather than impulse. By combining balanced nutrition, proper hydration, timely rituals, and brief movement, you keep your momentum through day 21 and beyond.

DIGESTIVE COMFORT & WHEN TO SEEK HELP

During your 21-day pink salt challenge, you may notice changes in digestion—some welcome, others less so. A gentle increase in bowel regularity, reduced bloating, or fewer gas episodes can accompany improved hydration and mineral balance. Yet for some, introducing pink salt and the accompanying dietary shifts may trigger discomfort: cramping, irregular movements, or a feeling of heaviness. Understanding how pink salt impacts digestion, identifying when small tweaks will help, and knowing when professional support is needed ensures you stay comfortable and confident throughout your journey.

How Pink Salt Affects Digestion

Pink salt contains sodium and chloride—key electrolytes that draw water into the digestive tract, aiding stool passage and preventing constipation. When you sip your morning elixir, you prime your intestines with fluid, stimulating motility. Better hydration also helps break down food particles, enhancing nutrient absorption in the small intestine. At the same time, pink salt's trace minerals—magnesium, potassium, and calcium—support muscle contractions lining the digestive tract, smoothing the wave-like movements (peristalsis) that move food along.

However, sudden increases in sodium can lead to temporary water retention in the gut wall, causing a sensation of bloating. If your overall fluid intake doesn't rise alongside added pink salt, you may experience harder stools or infrequent bowel movements. Similarly, if your fiber intake shifts dramatically—say, swapping refined grains for larger servings of vegetables—you might notice gas or cramping as gut bacteria adjust to new substrates. Recognizing these normal adaptation phases helps you distinguish between transient discomfort and signals warranting adjustments.

Simple Adjustments for Comfort

If you experience mild bloating, cramping, or irregularity, try these practical strategies:

- Increase water intake by an extra 8–16 ounces per day to match the osmotic pull of added sodium.
- Spread your pink salt dose over two servings—half in the morning, half mid-afternoon—to avoid a single high-sodium load.
- Balance fiber gradually: if you've doubled your vegetable portions, add an extra serving of beans or cabbage one meal at a time rather than all at once.
- Include gentle movement after meals—five minutes of walking or light stretching can stimulate digestion without pressure.
- Consider digestive aids like a slice of ginger or a teaspoon of apple cider vinegar in water before meals to activate digestive enzymes.

When Luz, a busy accountant, began her pink salt routine, she noticed bloating after lunch. By splitting her salt dose and adding a midday glass of water with lemon, her discomfort subsided in three days.

Recognizing Warning Signs

Most digestive changes during this challenge are temporary. Yet certain signs indicate that you should slow down, adjust more substantially, or consult a professional:

- Painful cramping that does not ease with hydration or movement.
- Persistent diarrhea lasting more than 24 hours, risking dehydration.
- Blood in stool or black, tarry bowel movements, which suggest bleeding.
- Unintentional weight loss exceeding five percent of body weight in two weeks.
- Severe or unexplained nausea and vomiting, preventing you from keeping fluids down.

If you encounter these symptoms, stop experimenting with pink salt adjustments until you've assessed your overall diet and hydration. Keep a log of foods, fluids, and symptoms, and share it with a healthcare provider if issues persist.

When to Seek Professional Support

Occasional tweaks at home can fix most discomforts, but chronic or severe symptoms require expert input. Suppose you've tried increasing fluids, balancing fiber, and adjusting salt timing for a week, yet you're still experiencing significant bloating or irregularity. In that case, you may have an underlying issue—irritable bowel syndrome, fructose intolerance, or a malabsorption disorder—that needs targeted treatment.

Connecting with a registered dietitian can help you personalize your plan: they can test for food sensitivities, design a feeding schedule, and suggest probiotic or enzyme supplements. A gastroenterologist can perform diagnostics like blood tests, stool analysis, or imaging to rule out conditions such as inflammatory bowel disease or gallbladder dysfunction. Timely evaluation ensures you continue the pink salt ritual safely and effectively.

Supporting Long-Term Digestive Health

As you move beyond day 21, aim to build digestive resilience into your daily routine:

- Maintain balanced hydration—continue sipping pink salt elixirs or move to natural mineral water if you prefer gradual reduction.
- Include fermented foods—yogurt, kimchi, or kefir—to nurture healthy gut flora alongside your ritual.
- Practice mindful eating—chew slowly, pause between bites, and notice fullness cues to avoid overloading your system.
- Keep a simple symptom journal—note any digestive changes as your diet evolves seasonally or with new recipes.

By integrating these habits, you lay the groundwork for ongoing comfort and vitality. Digestive comfort isn't a static goal but a dynamic balance between what you eat, how you hydrate, and how you listen to your body.

CHAPTER 9

Maintenance & Next Steps

TRANSITIONING TO LONG-TERM RITUALS

Moving beyond the initial 21 days of your pink salt challenge means weaving elements of your ritual into everyday life. The goal is not to maintain rigid steps forever but to adopt habits that feel natural and sustainable. As you build on the momentum of your first three weeks, consider which parts of the ritual brought you the greatest benefits—whether that was increased energy, smoother digestion, or steadier appetite—and explore ways to integrate them into varying routines, whether on workdays, weekends, or holidays.

Identifying Core Elements to Sustain

Not every step from day one needs permanent adoption. Reflect on your experience: did taking pink salt at sunrise ignite your morning focus? Did tracking your water intake keep cravings at bay? Pinpoint the practices that delivered the most value.

- Morning elixir timing that aligned with your work start and gave you 30 minutes of clear-headed productivity.
- A brief mid-afternoon hydration break with pink salt to prevent the slump before your final meeting.
- Routine tracking of energy and mood that revealed patterns in your sleep and nutrition choices.

By cataloging which actions had the strongest impact—whether 10 minutes of journaling, a glass of pink salt water, or a short walk—you can prioritize preserving those in your weekly rhythm and let go of extras that felt burdensome.

Adapting Rituals to Daily Life

Life rarely follows a fixed schedule. Weekdays, you might rise at 6:00 a.m.; weekends, you sleep later. Vacations, work events, or travel can disrupt your pattern. To transition smoothly, build variations of your ritual:

Flexible Timing

Rather than anchoring the elixir exclusively to "upon waking," connect it to consistent cues:

- When you turn off your alarm or first check your phone.
- Immediately after brushing your teeth or stepping into the shower.
- At the top of each hour during a morning block of focused work.

This way, if you sleep in or change zones, you can still trigger the habit without guilt.

Alternative Formats

On days when you're racing to a meeting or on the road, having grab-and-go options keeps you on course:

- Pre-mix single servings of pink salt in portable pouches to add to bottled water.
- Use a small stainless-steel bottle with measured markings to hold the water-plus-salt mix the night before.
- Swap the elixir for a mineral-rich tea infusion—hibiscus or green tea—when you need caffeine but still want electrolytes.

These substitutes maintain the ritual's function—hydration, mineral balance, and focus—without demanding extra preparation.

Integrating New Habits Gradually

Once the pink salt ritual feels stable, begin layering other healthy habits without overwhelming yourself. The first three weeks taught you how small changes lead to big effects; use that principle for next steps.

- Add one new recipe from your challenge each week, rotating ingredients to match produce availability and seasonality.
- Introduce a brief gratitude or intention-setting exercise at the end of your morning ritual to foster a positive mindset.
- Experiment with a weekly "dry run" day—skip other added supplements or routines to test which habits you truly miss.

By adding one habit at a time, you ensure each has room to integrate and stick rather than create a pile-up of tasks.

Case Example: From Challenge to Lifestyle

Consider Jenna, a marketing director who completed the 21-day pink salt program last summer. She loved the afternoon elixir for quelling energy dips and the daily recipe rotations that expanded her cooking skills. To maintain this:

1. She switched her morning ritual to "after coffee" rather than "after sunrise," accommodating her shift to hybrid work.
2. She pre-packed pink salt sachets in her tote, ensuring she never missed the 3 p.m. elixir, even during client visits.
3. Each Sunday, she chose two new recipes—one breakfast and one snack—to feature during the week, keeping variety without overhauling her meal plan.
4. She continued tracking energy levels in a small notebook until she felt confident recognizing patterns without logging every day.

Jenna's evolving ritual fit her 9-to-5, travel days, and weekend routines, making her feel supported rather than restricted by the process.

Avoiding Over-Ritualization

A long-term ritual should enhance life, not become a source of stress. If you find yourself obsessing over perfect timing or feeling guilty when you skip a step, it's time to simplify. Ask:

- Can I combine two steps into one, such as pairing intention-setting with my hydration break?
- Is there a core benefit I'm chasing, like hydration, that I can achieve through simpler means—plain water or electrolyte-rich foods?
- What's the minimum viable ritual that still keeps me feeling the benefits without micromanaging every detail?

Refining your approach keeps rituals sustainable and enjoyable rather than burdensome chores.

By choosing core elements to carry forward, adapting timing and format to your life's rhythms, integrating new habits one at a time, and streamlining when necessary, you ensure that the pink salt ritual becomes a flexible framework for lasting vitality rather than a fleeting 21-day experiment.

ADVANCED RECIPE ROTATIONS & SEASONAL SWAPS

As you move into maintenance after day 21, embracing variety through advanced recipe rotations and seasonal swaps keeps your meals exciting, maximizes nutrient intake, and aligns your pink salt ritual with nature's rhythms. Rather than repeating the same recipes each week, building a flexible framework of rotating themes and ingredient seasons ensures you never get bored and continually tap into fresh produce at its peak.

Establishing Rotation Cycles

Rotation isn't random—it follows a simple structure to balance familiarity with novelty. Start by grouping recipes into categories: breakfasts, lunches, dinners, snacks, and beverages. Within each category, create three subgroups. For example, breakfast might include smoothies, grain-based bowls, and egg-centered dishes. Each week, choose one subgroup per category:

- Week one: smoothies, grain bowls, egg dishes.
- Week two: overnight oats, frittatas, elixirs with add-ins like ginger or lemon.
- Week three: pancakes, parfaits, savory toasts.

This pattern ensures every recipe returns every three weeks—enough time to keep it fresh without completely abandoning dishes you enjoy.

Mapping Seasonal Ingredients

Aligning your recipes with seasonal produce not only supports local farming but also offers optimal flavor and nutrition. Seasonal swaps adjust your rotation based on what's abundant:

Spring

- Leafy greens—spinach, arugula, and ramps—appear in salads and pesto for lunches and dinners.
- Asparagus, peas, and rhubarb feature in side dishes and desserts, paired with pink salt to highlight their sweetness.
- Herbs like chives, parsley, and mint boost snacks and elixirs with bright aromatics.

Summer

- Berries—strawberries, blueberries, raspberries—for smoothies, parfaits, and fruit salad cups, drizzled with pink salt and lemon.
- Tomatoes, zucchini, and cucumbers star in cold soups and grilled skewers, seasoned with pink salt and fresh herbs.
- Mango, watermelon, and stone fruits create refreshing beverages and elixirs enhanced by a pinch of pink salt.

Fall

- Root vegetables—sweet potatoes, beets, carrots—in grain bowls and roasted veggie sides with pink salt and rosemary.
- Pumpkin, apples, and pears in breakfasts like porridge or pancakes spiced with cinnamon and pink salt.

- Kale and Swiss chard in soups, stir-fries, and frittatas, adding hearty greens as the temperature cools.

Winter

- Citrus—oranges, grapefruits, lemons—for invigorating elixirs and salads to counter the gray months.
- Cruciferous vegetables—broccoli, cauliflower, Brussels sprouts—roasted or stir-fried with pink salt and garlic.
- Squash and root mash dishes enriched with pink salt and nutmeg for warming dinners.

By syncing your recipe rotation with each season's bounty, you maximize nutrient diversity, cost savings, and flavor.

Building an Advanced Recipe Matrix

To manage this complexity, create a simple matrix combining rotation cycles and seasonal swaps. On a chart, list weeks horizontally and categories vertically. Fill each cell with specific recipes or ingredients based on season. At a glance, you see exactly which recipes to prepare, minimizing decision fatigue.

- Create a spreadsheet or whiteboard with columns for Week 1, Week 2, and Week 3, repeating every quarter.
- Under "Lunch," list three recipes per rotation, each tagged with seasonal produce—for example, "Spring Pea & Pink Salt Soup" in April and "Summer Zoodle Salad" in July.
- Update the matrix quarterly to reflect shifting seasons and include new recipes discovered through experimentation or community sharing.

This matrix becomes your culinary roadmap—clear, flexible, and visually engaging.

Case Study: Seasonal Swap in Action

Alex, a school teacher, found herself repeatedly cooking the same summer dishes year after year. By implementing a recipe matrix, she built a three-week rotation: breakfasts (smoothie bowl, chia pudding, frittata), lunches (quinoa salad, veggie wrap, grain bowl), dinners (stir-fry, soup, roast). Each quarter, she mapped seasonal swaps. In spring, her lunch rotation featured asparagus wraps and pea soup; in fall, she moved to pumpkin grain bowls and beet salads. The system kept her excited to cook, prevented grocery waste, and deepened her connection to local farmers' markets.

Through these structured yet adaptable rotations and swaps, you preserve the benefits of your pink salt ritual—steady energy, balanced nutrition, and a sense of novelty—while avoiding the trap of meal monotony. This approach lets you enjoy the full spectrum of nature's flavors and nutrients, season after season, as part of a long-term, sustainable lifestyle.

BUILDING COMMUNITY & ACCOUNTABILITY

Changing how you eat and hydrate can feel isolating without support. Yet when you tap into a community and create accountability systems, you gain motivation, fresh ideas, and a sense of shared purpose. Whether you connect with friends in person or join an online group, building community around your pink salt ritual turns a solo challenge into a shared adventure, making you more likely to stick with healthier habits long term.

Finding or Forming Your Community

Your circle might include friends, family, coworkers, or fellow pink salt enthusiasts online. Seek connections that balance encouragement with real-world perspectives:

- Invite a friend or colleague to commit to a 21-day challenge together, sharing weekly check-ins over coffee or video chat.
- Look for local wellness meetups—running clubs, cooking workshops, or nutrition seminars—where you can introduce the pink salt ritual and find others pursuing better hydration and balance.
- Join social media groups or forums dedicated to healthy living, weight loss, or natural remedies; share your progress and swap recipes and troubleshooting tips.

When Rebecca, a busy teacher, joined a weekend farmers' market cooking demo, she met two neighbors also experimenting with pink salt. They formed a weekly potluck group, rotating recipes from the challenge and offering each other feedback on tweaks and outcomes.

Establishing Accountability Structures

Accountability gives you a gentle nudge on days when motivation wanes. Effective systems combine regular check-ins, goal reminders, and shared record-keeping:

- Schedule brief weekly meetings—15 minutes—to discuss energy levels, recipe successes, and any plateaus or challenges.
- Create a shared digital tracker—using a simple spreadsheet or an app like Google Sheets—where each person logs their pink salt intake, energy rating, and one lesson learned that week.
- Set up automated reminders on your phone or calendar to take your pink salt elixir, record measurements, or prepare recipes.

Accountability works best when expectations are clear but flexible. Agree as a group to respect each other's pace—some may need to adjust sodium doses more gradually, others may prefer added movement rituals.

Encouragement Through Shared Stories

Reading or hearing about others' transformations provides both inspiration and practical tips. Encourage community members to share:

- Before-and-after anecdotes—how their energy, sleep, or cravings changed over the three weeks.
- Favorite recipe discoveries and how they adapted ingredients for allergies or preferences.
- Unexpected benefits—more restful sleep, boosted mood, or reduced digestive discomfort.

Hearing that Carlos, a father of two, overcame midday energy crashes by splitting his pink salt into two smaller doses gave others permission to personalize timing rather than feeling they had to follow the plan exactly.

Peer Support for Troubleshooting

When questions arise—how to manage sodium during travel, what to do on cheat days, or how to adjust when you hit a plateau—having peers to brainstorm with speeds solutions:

- Use group chat or thread discussions to post questions and receive multiple perspectives within hours.
- Organize mini "hackathons" where each member brings a challenge faced that week and the group collaborates on three possible tweaks.
- Rotate the role of weekly "challenge guru," responsible for gathering a new tip or research tidbit to share with the group.

This collaborative problem-solving builds collective knowledge and reminds you that plateaus or discomforts are normal, not personal failures.

Celebrating Milestones Together

Marking progress sustains momentum. Plan group celebrations for key milestones:

- Host a healthy brunch when the group completes the 21-day challenge, featuring favorite recipes from the book.
- Create digital badges or certificates for reaching benchmarks—seven days consistent, logging every day, or trying all four recipe chapters.
- Share small rewards—digital gift cards to a local health food store or free pass to a yoga class—for members who demonstrate creativity or perseverance.

Celebrations reinforce positive behavior and strengthen the social bonds that underlie accountability.

Extending Beyond the Initial Challenge

A strong community evolves past day 21 into an ongoing network of support:

- Form subgroups for maintenance goals—one for recipe rotations, another for fitness challenges, and another for mindful eating discussions.
- Plan quarterly cooking nights where each member teaches a new seasonal recipe from the pink salt framework.
- Annual check-ins around the same calendar dates to reflect on progress, set fresh goals, and renew commitment to rituals that still serve your health.

By weaving community and accountability into daily life, you transform the pink salt ritual from a one-time experiment into a lifestyle supported by shared experience, mutual encouragement, and a collective quest for better health.

TRACKING BEYOND DAY 21: TOOLS & TEMPLATES

Keeping momentum after your initial 21-day pink salt ritual relies on tracking progress and staying organized. Whether you prefer digital solutions or printable sheets, choosing the right tools and templates helps you maintain healthy habits, spot trends, and make adjustments when needed. Below are strategies and examples to build a tracking system that fits your lifestyle and keeps you engaged.

Digital Tools for Seamless Monitoring

Apps and online platforms offer automated reminders, data visualization, and device syncing. Consider these options:

- Habit-tracking apps such as Habitica or Streaks allow you to create recurring check-ins for your pink salt elixir, water intake, and daily recipe choices. They provide visual streaks and simple dashboards to celebrate consistency.
- Nutrition trackers like MyFitnessPal or Cronometer can log your sodium intake automatically as you enter meals. You can add a custom food entry for your pink salt drink to track its contribution to your daily electrolyte goals.
- Spreadsheet templates in Google Sheets or Excel give you complete control over the metrics you record. Set up columns for date, time of elixir, fluid ounces consumed, energy rating (1–5), notes on cravings or digestion, and recipe of the day. Use built-in charts to spot weekly trends and correlations.

When you sync your tracker with a wearable device—such as a Fitbit or Apple Watch—you can integrate activity, sleep, and heart-rate data. This holistic view helps you see how hydration, nutrition, and movement interact, guiding you to tweak timing or dosage for optimal results.

Printable Templates for Hands-On Journaling

If you find digital tools distracting, a paper approach may suit you better. Printable templates combine structure with the tactile pleasure of writing:

- A daily log sheet with sections for morning elixir time, water intake tally, mood/energy levels at three checkpoints (morning, midday, evening), and space for brief observations. Keep it on your bedside table or kitchen counter for easy access.
- A weekly overview page that lists each day of the week down the left margin and tracks recipe rotations, community check-in notes, and hydration targets. Use symbols—like a dot for completed elixir and a dash for skipped—to glance at your adherence pattern.
- A monthly summary worksheet where you total your "days elixir taken," average energy score, number of recipe experiments, and any acute symptoms such as cravings or plateaus. Color-code highs and lows to visualize which weeks felt strongest and which might need adjustments.

Laminate key templates or place them in a binder so you can use a dry-erase marker for ongoing tracking. This keeps your system low-cost and environmentally friendly.

Customizing Templates for Your Needs

No single template fits everyone. Tailor yours based on what matters most:

- If digestion is a focus, include a brief "digestive comfort" rating scale and space for notes on bloating or regularity.
- For those who jog or cycle, add a column for workout type and duration, then annotate whether your pink salt timing affected muscle cramps or endurance.
- When community support is key, incorporate a "peer check-in" checkbox and line for feedback received or given each week, reinforcing accountability.

Adjust column widths and line spacing for readability. You might start with a daily sheet, realize you only need three times per week logging, and switch to a simplified tracker. Flexibility ensures you only record what you'll actually maintain.

Integrating Reminders & Automation

Whether digital or analog, reminders keep your system alive:

- Use phone alarms or calendar events to prompt your morning and afternoon elixirs. Label them with short encouragements—"Time for your pink salt boost!"—to spark motivation.
- Set monthly recurring tasks to review your logs, perhaps on the first of each month, so you don't let weeks slip by without reflection.
- In a paper journal, place sticky-note reminders on your bathroom mirror or fridge door to nudge you before meal prep or bedtime.

By automating these cues, you reduce reliance on willpower alone and embed tracking into your daily environment.

Reviewing and Refining Your System

Regular review sessions consolidate your insights into action steps:

- Every two weeks, spend 10 minutes with your tracker summarizing what worked—stable energy, reduced cravings—and where adjustments are needed—bloating, missed elixirs.
- Use a simple "start, stop, continue" framework: start any new habit (like a gratitude note), stop a redundant step (perhaps daily logs if weekly suffice), and continue the core elements that yield the biggest payoff.
- Share summaries with your accountability group or a coach to celebrate successes and brainstorm solutions for lingering challenges.

This iterative cycle of tracking, reviewing, and refining keeps your pink salt ritual responsive to changing life demands and health goals.

By leveraging digital apps for automation, printable templates for tactile engagement, customizable fields for personalization, and structured review sessions, you create a robust tracking framework that extends beyond day 21. Such a system grounds your long-term efforts in data, self-reflection, and community support, ensuring the habits you've built continue to nurture your vitality.

Conclusion

Over the past weeks, you've embarked on a simple yet powerful ritual: a daily pink salt elixir to kick-start your hydration and metabolism; carefully chosen recipes that nourish your body and delight your senses; practical tracking tools that turn impressions into insights; and a supportive structure that adapts to the ebb and flow of your life. What began as an experiment has grown into a living practice designed to meet you where you are—whether juggling meetings and carpools, snatching moments between emails, or carving out quiet minutes before the day's rush. Along the way, you've learned that real change isn't born from extremes but from consistent, intentional steps that honor your unique rhythms.

Perhaps most surprising is how much this journey hinges on connection—connection to your body's subtle signals, to traditions that reach back through centuries, and to a community of fellow challengers cheering you on. When you stirred that first glass of pink salt water, you were tapping into an ancient practice. Yet each time you measured your waist, logged your energy, or reflected on cravings, you rewrote the script for what routine could mean: not a chore but a chance to learn, adapt, and grow. Those daily notes in your journal, the checkmarks on your habit tracker, and even the occasional missed day served as data points, guiding you toward what works and signaling where to fine-tune.

You've seen how a quarter teaspoon of mineral-rich salt can transform more than a drink. It can steady your mood, sharpen your focus, and help your cells draw in water and nutrients more efficiently. By pairing that ritual with thoughtfully designed recipes—each balanced for flavor, texture, and the pink salt principle—you've given your metabolism the tools it needs to favor fat oxidation over sugar crashes. Morning elixirs set the tone for afternoons without energy slumps; smartly seasoned meals kept sodium in check while delivering trace minerals; and snacks offered satisfying crunches that quieted cravings without derailing your progress.

But beyond the science of electrolytes and fat-burning, you've embraced a mindset shift: that self-care can be practical, even playful, woven seamlessly into your busy life. You learned how to adapt the plan for travel days by packing salt sachets and a reusable bottle, and how to honor your ritual during late shifts by reimagining "morning" as the first moment you're awake. You discovered the power of habit stacking—attaching your new action to a familiar cue—and how portable tracking tools kept motivation high, even when your calendar flipped upside down.

Along this path, you've also navigated plateaus, those inevitable moments when the scale stalls or waist measurements hold steady. Instead of seeing them as failures, you reframed plateaus as invitations to revisit your data, examine your sleep, hydration, sodium intake, and even stress levels. Maybe you realized that weekend celebrations needed simpler snack swaps or that adding a pinch of lemon or ginger to your elixir offered both flavor and digestive support. Each adjustment reaffirmed that lasting progress unfolds in small increments, guided by your own observations and curiosity.

By Day 21, you may have lost a few pounds or inches, or perhaps you simply experienced steadier energy and fewer cravings. Those concrete wins are satisfying, yet the deeper reward lies in the confidence you've built—that you can set a clear goal, track meaningful metrics, and respond when life shifts rather than abandoning the effort. You've learned to celebrate micro-wins: a week of consistent hydration, a recipe that curbed afternoon hunger, or a morning where you resisted mindless snacking. These victories stacked to form a foundation for habits that outlast any single challenge.

Looking ahead, the 21-day framework fades into the background, but the practices remain. You might still begin—or end—your day with that rosy pinch of salt, now second nature. You'll rotate recipes seasonally, swapping strawberries for squash, mint for rosemary, but you'll carry the same principles: balanced electrolytes, mindful flavor, and simple preparation. You'll continue to track key markers when you need a course correction—perhaps before a big event or after a period of travel—but you'll also trust the rhythms you've built, knowing when to lean in and when to rest.

Above all, this journey underscores one truth: genuine wellbeing emerges from consistency, not perfection. You've proven that even in the busiest seasons—amid deadlines, school runs, and family gatherings—a small ritual can anchor your intentions and yield real benefits. You've seen how ancient wisdom, modern science, and personal experimentation converge in a single pinch of salt. And you've discovered that the most meaningful transformations occur when you treat your body with curiosity and kindness, listening to its feedback and adjusting with compassion.

As you close this chapter and step forward, remember that every glass you stir, every recipe you savor, and every data point you record is part of a larger conversation with yourself. Keep that dialogue alive. Share your story with others, invite a friend to try the ritual, or simply revisit your notes when you need a reminder of how far you've come. Change rarely happens in leaps and bounds; it unfolds in the everyday choices you repeat until they become your new normal.

Your pink salt challenge may be complete, but your journey continues. Carry forward the lessons you've learned—the power of small habits, the importance of consistency, and the joy of tuning into your body's needs. In those moments when you taste that gentle saltiness, pause and appreciate the ritual you've mastered. Each sip becomes a bridge between where you were and where you're headed, a reminder that wellness is crafted one deliberate choice at a time.

Unlock Your Free Pink Salt Bonuses!

Get instant access to two powerful tools designed to streamline your ritual and amplify your results:

21-Day Pink Salt Challenge Journal

Your interactive PDF companion for daily elixir logs, energy ratings, mood notes, and weekly reflections.

Seasonal Shopping & Meal-Prep Guide

A four-season toolkit with produce pairings, tick-list shopping sheets, and ready-made meal plans.

Scan the QR code now to download both PDFs—and keep your momentum strong!

Printed in Dunstable, United Kingdom